FOOD AND SOCIETY

FOOD

AND SOCIETY

Magnus Pyke

JOHN MURRAY
FIFTY ALBEMARLE STREET LONDON

TX
357
P95

© Magnus Pyke 1968
First published 1968
Reprinted 1971

Printed Offset Litho in Great Britain
for John Murray (Publishers) Ltd
by Cox & Wyman Ltd, London
Fakenham and Reading
0 7195 1801 6

CONTENTS

FOREWORD

The theme of this book is that there is more to nutrition than what is usually taught as nutrition. People eat food, they do not ingest nutrients. Nutrition is, to be sure, a special aspect of biochemistry which itself sprang from physiology. But these are all aspects of biology, the science of living things, which itself comprehends anthropology, the study of man. A conventional training in nutritional science is an insufficient guide to those who feel moved to change the social habits and religious customs of distant communities. Nor is technical advice on agriculture and contraception of itself guaranteed to change the traditional customs of ancient peoples. Besides which, anthropology is not only concerned with remote races and their strange customs: we too have irrational antipathies and beliefs, and are gullible and superstitious in spite of our scientific virtuosity. Our anthropological peculiarities are often revealed, just as are those of other races, in our eating habits and our attitudes to foods of various kinds.

It is instructive and at times grotesquely amusing to study what man eats and why, and to what extent nutrition is the main motive for his dietary behaviour. Often it is difficult to disentangle the facts from the fallacies in pursuing such studies. If, however, my fellow nutritionists may be brought to question some of their basic assumptions by reading this book, and if those who are seeking to know what nutrition is about and thus improve the state of needy communities may come to see how subtle are the reactions between what people eat and what else they do, I shall have succeeded in my purpose.

MAGNUS PYKE

vii

CHAPTER I

NOT BY BREAD ALONE

The science of nutrition, as it is understood and practised today, is the fruit of a century of revolutionary intellectual activity. During the Industrial Revolution, Western people had quite suddenly got the idea of combining scientific principles, which had been growing as ideas since the great times of Newton, Boyle and Galileo in the seventeenth century, with technology. The centre and motive force was the steam engine. In the latter part of the nineteenth century, seized with the euphoria of technological progress, people began to devote themselves to science in the way we do now, not so much from the love of scholarship and the desire to unlock the secrets of nature, but to be useful. With a rush, chemistry assumed its modern form and, to a very large degree, made physiology and medicine possible. It was Pasteur, a chemist, who almost single-handed 'invented' bacteriology and the germ theory of disease in the middle decades of the century.

Almost the whole of nutritional science, in its current form, has grown in little more than the last sixty years. It is true that in the nineteenth century a number of chemists carried out analysis on diets, and separated the components of foods into the broad classifications now called carbohydrates, fats and proteins. But it did not require any very sophisticated chemistry to discover that meat is made up of two very different substances; the fat, and the lean or protein part. Nor did it require very profound science to distinguish that starch, whether derived from flour, rice or potato, was different again from both. The 'newer knowledge of nutrition' as E. V. McCollum[1] called it later on, started when C. A. Pekelharing, Professor of Hygiene in the University of Utrecht, published the results of his feeding experiments on mice in 1905.[2] These were a model of the precise controlled study carried out on a narrow, well-defined front; such studies, in the hands of his successors, led to the rapid advances which built up the massive corpus of today's nutritional orthodoxy.

[1] McCollum, E. V., *The Newer Knowledge of Nutrition*, 1918.
[2] Pekelharing, C. A., *Nederlandsch Tij. N. Geneesk*, 2, 3, 1905.

Pekelharing fed mice a diet composed of casein, the protein of milk, mixed with egg white, together with rice flour as a source of carbohydrate and lard to supply fat. In addition, he added a mixture of such mineral components as had been found to be of physiological importance. It was a limited but – in the terms of 1905 – scientifically 'balanced' diet. At first the mice thrived, but soon they began to lose their appetite, and within four weeks all of them had died. Pekelharing collected a second group of mice and fed them the same diet, adding a ration of milk. The mice did not lose their appetite but remained alive and well. Even when a third group received only whey as a supplement in place of milk, they remained well. Pekelharing deduced that there was an unknown substance in the milk and in the whey essential to the nutritional wellbeing of mice.

It is a historical oddity that the work of Pekelharing, like that of the Abbé Johann Mendel before him, was overlooked for a number of years and for the same reason – that it was published in a journal not widely read. And so, in 1912, Hopkins[3] working in Cambridge achieved considerable renown for very much the same experiment, but done with rats instead of mice. Only in 1926 was Pekelharing's work discovered by English-speaking scientists. But by then Casimir Funk[4] had invented the term 'vitamins' to describe the unknown substances whose presence was necessary for the proper nutrition of men as well as rodents.

The exact chemical composition of vitamins did not remain unknown long. Their elucidation was ideally suited to the intellectual climate of the scientific age. Rats fed a certain synthetic diet became frowsy and ill. Their fur grew 'staring' and untidy, and looked unhealthy; young ones ceased to grow; their eyes discharged pus and became bloodshot. Before long the infected corneas of their eyeballs, afflicted by xerophthalmia, perforated and the animals became blind. When cod-liver oil was added to their diet none of this happened. When the cod-liver oil was divided into its chemical components and the fatty part separated from the so-called non-saponifiable fraction, it was the latter which was found to possess the preventive action. Soon, following a systematic series of separations, each tested for its physiological effect on a group of rats, the pure substance, active when added to the diet in very small measured amounts, was identi-

[3] Hopkins, F. G., *J. Physiol.*, 44, 425, 1912.
[4] Funk, C., *J. State Med.*, 20, 341, 1912.

fied. And as for young rats, so it was for young human beings. In 1917 Professor C. E. Bloch[5] published his account of the children in Copenhagen afflicted by xerophthalmia. During World War I, food science had enabled the manufacture of margarine to replace the Danish butter, and it was exported to the Allies and the Central Powers alike; but allowance was not made for the existence of the newly identified 'accessory food factor', vitamin A. Harsh experience showed that this vitamin A-deficiency affected children just as it did rats. An adequate diet, it could now be seen, included in addition to its carbohydrate, protein, fat and mineral components, a measured amount of vitamin A as well.

Each of a series of 'accessory food factors' was discovered, identified, its physiological action investigated and the quantity needed for health estimated. The chemistry of one B-vitamin, riboflavin, was worked out in 1933; that of another, thiamine, in 1936; and that of a third, niacin, in 1937. The elucidation of the chemical composition of vitamin C, the antiscurvy vitamin, was finally established in 1933. Although the Scottish surgeon, James Lind,[6] had carried out chemical trials at sea in 1747 clearly showing that oranges contained a substance which would cure scurvy, the discovery of what the nature of the substance was, and how much of it was needed for the maintenance of health, had to wait nearly 200 years. The attack of the modern scientific method quickly revealed the facts: for instance, it was found that rats and mice could not be used as test animals, since, by a biochemical anomaly, these animals do not need vitamin C in their diet.

A massive collection of accurate knowledge has accrued during the early decades of the twentieth century, and the importance of the scientific work that has been done cannot be minimized. In many instances, not only have nutritional factors causing disease been detected and their precise chemical configuration elucidated, but their biochemical mechanisms in the living tissues have been discovered as well. Thus it was a great triumph to discover that such diseases as pellagra and beri-beri, which continuously scourged tropical countries, are due not to the presence of a pathogenic microorganism as are typhus or yellow fever, but rather to the absence of a necessary dietary component. More profound, however, was the

[5] Bloch, C. E., *Ugeskrift*, f. Laeger, 79, 349, 1917.
[6] Lind, J., *A Treatise on the Scurvy*, 1753.

understanding of how the absent factors – thiamine in beri-beri and niacin in pellagra – fit into the harmonious working of the cells of well-nourished individuals. By studying the effect of vitamins not only in human tissues and in those of experimental animals, but also in the growth and reproduction of lower creatures – insects, yeasts or bacteria – the diverse biochemistry of different species has been illuminated. More important still has been the finding that within this diversity there is an underlying unity. Perhaps one of the greatest scientific achievements of a century of work has been the conception of the uniformity of the life process as a whole.

Arising from this confident and well-consolidated scientific advance, lists of nutrients have been prepared by expert bodies – by the League of Nations, the Food and Nutrition Board of the US National Research Council, the British Medical Association, the authorities in Canada, in India and wherever scientific work is done. Latest of all, the Food and Agriculture Organization and the World Health Organization of the United Nations have consolidated the nutritional science of the world. All these tables of recommended nutritional intake set out in exact quantitative terms the amount of this vitamin or that, of calcium, iron or iodine, of one amino-acid component of protein or another which, on average, a man (sedentary or engaged in heavy labour), a woman (pregnant or not), or a child of a given age, must eat for nutritional wellbeing.[7]

Those who study nutritional science can be presented with a seemingly straightforward picture. They learn the values selected by the US National Research Council,[8] or the only marginally different figures of the British Medical Association[9] or FAO[10] of the requirement of adolescent girls, let us say, for phosphorus or cyanocobalamin. They can read the reports of experiments carried out on rats or hamsters, chickens or blackbeetles, providing the evidence upon which the official targets were based. They can also study accounts of children with rickets, of hunger oedema, or the heroic experiments of such a man as Crandon[11] who deprived himself of vitamin C and watched what happened to his own flesh. In the same tradition were

[7] Pyke, M., *Proc. VI Int. Congress Nutr.*, p. 54, Livingstone, 1964.
[8] USNRC., Food & Nutr. Board, Pub. 589, 1958.
[9] BMA., *Rept. of the Committee on Nutr.*, 1950.
[10] FAO., *Rept. 5*, 1950; *15*, 1957; *16*, 1957.
[11] Crandon, J. H., Lind, C. C., & Dill, D. B., *New Eng. J. Med.*, 223, 353, 1940.

the men who volunteered to suffer experimentally-induced starvation in Minneapolis, or vitamin A deficiency in Sheffield. The young scientist must learn the chemical composition of different foods, the effect on food composition – if any – of different methods of cultivation or of animal husbandry, the influence of cooking or of the processes of food technology. With all this in his head, the fully fledged nutritionist is ready to go out into the world and use his knowledge.

There are circumstances when the knowledge of nutrition so learned can be directly applied. The dreadful occurrence of rickets among the infants in Vienna at the end of World War I[12] was not repeated in World War II, because the chemistry of vitamin D (it is a sterol, calciferol, the formula of which can be written down by any competent biochemistry student) is understood, and its function in bone-formation known. But while the knowledge of scientific nutrition, set down in a dozen textbooks, enables anyone to assess whether or not the diet of a community is satisfactory and, if not, in what respect it must be remedied, there are many circumstances where the textbooks do not say how the situation can actually be remedied. This has required another line of research, into human behaviour, which has gone on parallel to the chemistry and the biochemistry.

In 1899, Seebohm Rowntree,[13] then a young man, carried out a detailed survey of the social conditions under which working-class families were living in the city of York. He found that many of them were suffering from extreme hardship: that their babies were dying, some of them from malnutrition. Some families, subsisting under conditions of approximately equal penury, contrived a little better. But he concluded that when the poverty of a family was sufficiently severe – and poverty was what they were all suffering from – there was a point when, no matter how wisely or frugally they managed their affairs, they could never procure for themselves an adequate diet, and would inevitably suffer from what could – with equal justice – be called either malnutrition or semi-starvation. Rowntree calculated in terms of money what he called his 'poverty line'. Families below it must be malnourished, he concluded, while those above it might have enough to eat if they had sufficient judgement to spend their money

12 Chick, H., & Dalzell, E. J., *Wien. Klin. Wschr.*, 32, 1219, 1919.
13 Rowntree, B. S., *Poverty: a study of town life*, Longmans, 1903.

wisely. He found that the 'standard death rate' of members of those families living below the poverty line was 27·8 per thousand whereas the rate for families with enough money to bring them above the line was 13·5. The effect of malnutrition is brought home more urgently by Rowntree's finding that, of every 1,000 babies born alive to families below the poverty line, 247 died before their first birthday. In households above the poverty line, out of each 1,000 babies 173 died.

In 1936, Seebohm Rowntree again surveyed the conditions of working-class families in York.[14] Prices of food had risen, but so had wages, and fewer people were found to be living under the poverty line. There still were some, but now their 'standardized death rate' was 13·5 compared with 8·4 for those above the line. Housing, sanitation and medical knowledge had advanced. And in 1936, 77·7 out of each 1,000 of the babies of the poorest parents died compared with 41·3 of those whose parents could afford a proper diet. This time it was possible to calculate from the figures collected in the survey which precise nutrients were lacking from the diets of the malnourished families. For example, those below the poverty line consumed only 52 per cent as much vitamin A as they needed for adequate health; above the line, the average amount available exceeded the requirement by 25 per cent.

The final astonishing achievement of Seebohm Rowntree, a remarkable man, was to complete a third survey of working-class families in York in 1950.[15] The increase in wealth had continued, the people had more money to spend, the numbers living below the poverty line were very few and, even so, their death rate was less, and fewer of their infant children died.

What does all this show? It shows first of all that when a community of people, as distinct from a colony of white rats imprisoned in cages, is suffering from nutritional deficiency, there are two ways of putting the matter right. A nutritional expert can analyse their diet to determine in what respect it is inadequate, whether in protein, vitamin A or iron; he can undertake clinical studies and biochemical analysis of specimens of blood and urine to confirm his deduction, and then he can add the necessary nutrients – casein as an addition to the bread, let us say, or vitamin A tablets for the expectant mothers,

[14] Rowntree, B. S., *Poverty and Progress*, Longmans, 1941.
[15] Rowntree, B. S., & Lavens, G. R., *Poverty and the Welfare State*, Longmans, 1951.

and iron as well. Alternatively, the nutritional wellbeing of the community can, as Rowntree's surveys show so vividly, be improved by supplying, not vitamins or minerals, but money. Furthermore, it is important for a wise nutritionist to know that, even if five shillings more a head is given to a family whose income is five shillings below the poverty line, it will not necessarily suffice to ensure an adequate diet. This is not the way people behave. They may spend part of their supplementary five shillings on food, they may even buy the right kind of food to enrich their diet in the correct nutrient. On the other hand, it is very likely that they will spend part of the money on cigarettes, or on a new dress for the eldest daughter or a pair of boots for father. Of all people, it is most important for a nutritional scientist, preoccupied as he will inevitably be by the intricacies of his speciality, to remember that man does not live by bread alone.

Take another example. Early in World War II, the British Government set to work seriously to apply scientific knowledge of nutrition to the feeding of the beleaguered population for which they were responsible. The total requirement of calories, of protein, fat, minerals and a dozen different vitamins was carefully calculated and set down on one side of a balance-sheet. On the other were listed the various food imports which it was hoped to bring into the country through the submarine blockade. Then there were the supplies for which home agriculture was to be responsible. These too were converted into terms of nutrients. Where the two sides of the sheet failed to balance, special steps were thought out. Vitamin C for babies and young children was made up by imports of concentrated orange-juice from abroad, supplemented by the collection of rose hips at home – especially those to be found in Scotland where the berries were discovered to be particularly rich in the vitamin – and the manufacture of a syrup from them. Vitamins A and D for expectant mothers were imported as capsules. Calcium for the population as a whole was, in the absence of enough cheese, provided by mixing chalk with the bread. The whole exercise was triumphantly justified by the well-maintained nutritional health of the population. Science was indeed vindicated; the increased wages of wartime, while they enabled families to buy nourishing foods, would have been unavailing by themselves had there not been sufficient of the right foods to buy.[16]

[16] Pyke, M., *Brit. Med. Bull.*, 2, 228, 1944.

One of the small points where things went wrong, however, was in the horticultural planning. Most of the land of the British Isles was devoted to corn, potatoes, dairy cattle, sheep on the high ground, and a limited number of pigs – limited because pigs may compete with people for the same foods. A special allotment of land was, however, set aside for vegetables. Of this, a certain area was to be devoted to the growing of cabbages, brussels-sprouts and spring greens, all good sources of vitamin C. Cauliflower could supply protein as well. Purple-sprouting broccoli would give a good yield of vitamins per acre at a time of year when fresh vegetables are scarce. Above all, the importance of devoting the allocated area of sandy soil to carrots was emphasized. Few other crops provide so many million international units of vitamin A-activity per acre. In this scientifically based nutritional plan for vegetables there was little room for onions, which contain only scanty amounts of recognized nutrients, and no room at all for gherkins.[17]

In planning the subsistence of an island community such as Great Britain for war, the maximum bulk of imports, and consequently the necessities for home production, needs to be decided. Then the carrying capacity of the available shipping must be judiciously allocated to the different kinds of imports. Wheat must compete for space with machinery, corned beef with spare parts for aeroplanes, eggs with radio sets. Each Department of State must argue its case with every other. And so it came about that when the Ministry of Food came to negotiate with the Ministry of War, the voice of the generals carried considerable weight. And one thing upon which the generals were adamant was, that there must be an adequate supply of gherkins. They were unmoved to learn from the nutritional experts that gherkins are – in terms of nutrients – of negligible significance. The British soldier, they insisted, could not fight without a proper supply of pickles to eat with his cold meat. And land was therefore allocated to grow the gherkins to make the pickles.

This is nutrition. The gherkin story exemplified two of its aspects. A living cell, or the great commonwealth of cells which together make up a human body, requires for its nourishment the list of proteins – or, rather, the selected amino acids of which the proteins are composed – and the fatty substances, the mineral salts and all the rest which are set down in the biochemical literature and tabulated in

[17] Pyke, M., *J. Amer. Dietetic Ass.*, 23, 90, 1947.

the nutritional recommendations of official commissioners. This is what the human body requires. But the human being to whom the body belongs does not necessarily see things in the same light.

What human communities choose to eat is only partly dependent on their physiological requirements, and even less on intellectual reasoning and a knowledge of what these physiological requirements are. Of equal significance is the complex psychological conditioning to which the individual and the group of which he is a member have been exposed. A curious mingling of reason, knowledge, superstition, and half-remembered wisdom of the tribe make up the corpus of food facts and fallacies which so-called educated, rational, twentieth-century people carry about in their heads. It is derived from many other sources than science. Consider, for example, the origin of fallacies.

CHAPTER II

FALLACIES

J. G. Frazer [1, 2], has described in detail the magic implications of food, and of eating and drinking. We, as scientific nutritionists, must still bear them in mind today: shared meals and State banquets even in the twentieth century possess a significance which is wider than that of the mere ingestion of nutrients. In many early societies it was believed that a man's enemy could do him harm if he gained possession of remains of food which he had eaten, and cast a spell on it. This belief had a strange result in Northern New Guinea, where all the cats have stumpy tails. This prevents their being stolen and eaten; the thief knows that their owner could cause him to fall ill by saying the necessary spell over the piece of cut-off tail, which is kept carefully in a safe place for this very contingency. Similarly, according to Frazer, the ancient Romans would immediately break the shells of the eggs or snails they had eaten to prevent ill-wishers making magic with them. Although the reason may now be lost, this custom – at least with egg-shells – can be found in our own society today. We retain a further residue of magic in feeling something of the moral bonds binding us in some small degree of good-will with people with whom we have a shared meal. As Frazer pointed out after studying diverse tribes, honour and good faith are strengthened by the fear of magic harm which could come to all those who have eaten together. No man would eat with another whom he proposed to injure by casting spells on the food leavings. If he did so he would, on the principles of sympathetic magic, suffer equally with his enemy. Both are united by the common food in their stomachs.

And modern dieticians must not lose patience when they find an undernourished wife giving the lion's share of meat to her husband to make him strong. This belief comes from remotest history. The

---

[1] Frazer, J. G., *The Golden Bough, Taboos and the Perils of the Soul*, Macmillan, N.Y., 1935.

[2] Frazer, J. G., *The Golden Bough, Spirits of the Corn and of the Wild*, II Macmillan, N.Y., 1935.

Abipones of Paraguay eat jaguars, bulls and stags to make them strong, brave and swift – and avoid eating hens and tortoises for fear of becoming cowardly and slow; the Miris of Assam prize tigers' flesh to make themselves fierce – but forbid it to their women; the Kansas Indians relish dogs' flesh on the grounds that by eating it they become brave and faithful. Caribs abstain from pigs' flesh lest their eyes become small, and the Aino people of Japan, who believe the otter to be a forgetful animal, refuse to eat it lest by so doing they lose their memory. These are just a few of the tribal beliefs about the magic of foods. We deceive ourselves if we forget that we too are heirs to such an inheritance just as are other communities. In a recent paper in the American Journal of Clinical Nutrition,[3] Moore drew attention to the fact that we accept food from friends and distrust what is offered by outsiders. This is abundantly apparent in the present age of easy foreign travel. Moore also pointed out that certain articles of diet – particularly meat – are considered to be masculine, and others feminine, regardless of the similarity in the nutritional needs of the two sexes. Yet another ethnological factor affecting eating is the use of special foods as badges of social status. Smoked salmon implies social superiority, cow heel and tripe are attributes of the lower castes.

The dogma of the West, which it is heresy to challenge, is that our dietary habits are based on reason: it is only remote foreign tribes which believe in taboos. We are brought up on the assumption that even Moses, when by a process of inspired intuition he forbade the Jews to eat pork, did so to protect their health. The basis for this belief is highly doubtful. The finding of pig bones in prehistoric and early historic sites from North Africa to the Indus Valley is evidence that pork was esteemed as a nutritious food from the earliest times. The quantity found at Tell Asmar suggests that pigs were probably the most important of all the domestic animals used by the Sumerians.[4] While for early medical evidence it is perhaps only necessary to quote Hippocrates who, somewhere around the year 460 BC, spoke of pork as providing more strength than other types of meat. Pork was also an important feature of every North East Chinese culture from the Neolithic onwards, and their use of vinegary sweet and sour

[3] Moore, H., *Amer. J. Chi. Nutr.* 5, 77, 1957.
[4] Hilyheimer, M., *Studies in Ancient Oriental Civilizations*, Chicago U.P., 20, 48, 1941.

sauce made the bones partly soluble, and thus provided useful calcium for pregnant mothers and their young children.

The modern 'scientific' argument that pork was forbidden because it can be the vehicle of the disease, trichinosis, is not at all convincing. The connection between infected pork and trichinosis is only a very recent discovery, and the link between the two is not at all obvious without up-to-date equipment. Other rather dubious evidence, which conventionally educated scientists know little about, is that, as the poet Hermesianax wrote in the fourth century BC, because a boar killed Attis the Phrygian, ever afterwards the Galatians abstained from pork. A more rational reason why some races forswear swine and support their rejection on religious grounds is that, since pigs cannot easily be herded over long distances, they are not popular among nomadic people – who then come to despise those more settled races who are able successfully to keep and eat pigs.

It may be said that nowadays we rational people, with our understanding of nutrition and of the world shortage of animal protein, do not allow ourselves to be influenced by such irrational matters as the mythical state of the hero Attis. Yet few Western nutritionists, no matter how clear-headed and rational, recommend the consumption of horseflesh, although in Belgium and France it is offered for sale. But the horse in Inner Asia even now serves the people for riding, the transport of goods, and the provision of milk, meat and hides. Landsell[5], writing in 1882 about the Yakut people in Siberia, describes how they preferred horsemeat to all other. Their favourite wedding dish was boiled horse's head served with horseflesh sausages. The most likely reason why Western dieticians feel a distaste for horse, in spite of the excellent quality of the protein of which it is mainly composed, has nothing at all to do with dietetics or for that matter with reason. Horsemeat eating was at one time a commonplace wherever horses were kept, from Mongolia all the way to Eastern Europe. Then, in the eighth century, Pope Gregory III ordered Boniface, his apostle to the Germans, to forbid the use of horseflesh by his Christian converts in order that they should show their separateness from the pagan tribes and vandals who ate wild horses and made a meal of horseflesh part of their pagan rites. And so there grew up in Christendom a belief that eating horses was wrong which persists to this day.

[5] Landsdell, H., *Through Siberia*, p. 811, Mefflin, 1882.

Since times of antiquity, dogflesh has been an esteemed article of diet in China. Indeed, the chow was specially bred for culinary purposes. Simoons[6] describes the preparation of puppy hams, and the use of suckling pups as delicacies. As far back as Neolithic times, dogs were eaten, and were second only to pigs in popularity: apart from their dietetic virtues, both were also valuable as scavengers. Both are also widely eaten in Africa, from Ghana and West Africa to the Congo, Nigeria, Angola and the Sudan. Why is it that although the views of so many people are quite permissive to the use of dogflesh as food, for most inhabitants of the industrial West the eating of dog is absolutely and violently taboo? The Polynesians eat dog. The Mbundu of Angola, just like the British, develop a strong affection for their dogs, nevertheless they eat and enjoy dogflesh. Is the antipathy of Western nations to eating dog related to Islamic views that they are 'unclean' carrion eaters, or must it be accepted as being entirely irrational?

The attribution of moral virtues to the consumption of certain foods or to abstinence from others derives, like magic, from the distant past. Apart from the rules of various religions, beliefs of almost theological intensity are to be found today in a variety of dietary systems. A significant number of people believe that foods prepared from crops manured with dung possess special virtues other than those measurable by scientific observation. The Pythagorean system required of its disciples abstinence from wine and from all animal food and recommended the use of such items as fruit, nuts, honey and milk which need no cooking. This doctrine has quite frequently been repeated in modern times. Oswald, writing in 1879,[7] refers to the Swiss system of 'Natur-Heilkunde' of a Dr Schrodt who claimed that the 'natural' foods for man are 'such vegetable and semi-animal products as either are or can be eaten and relished raw, and without the preliminaries of cooking and spicing'. Schrodt's system was most violently opposed to 'all ardent spices . . . and also those partly decayed and acid substances . . . strong cheese, sauerkraut and pickles'.

The gradual change of an idea initiated as an article of faith in the moral virtues of vegetarianism, let us say, or the vital qualities derived from the consumption of fertile eggs or so-called 'nature's'

6 Simoons, F. J., *Eat not this Flesh*, U. Wisconsin P., 1961.
7 Oswald, F. L., *Pop. Sci. Monthly*, 14, 721, 1879.

foods, into an allegedly rational dependence on scientific fact is a striking feature of many of the fallacies which have circulated during recent years. Undoubtedly, in nutrition a little learning is indeed a dangerous thing.

Dr Sylvester Graham was an American doctor of some note whose two-volume book, *Lectures on the Science of Life*, published in 1839[8] exerted a considerable influence on nutritional thought. So-called Graham bread and flour are still obtainable in the United States today. Mingled with certain sound observations on physiology, and supported by a good measure of clinical acumen, Graham's doctrine also included a remarkable infusion of emotional articles of faith, some of which clearly derived from the remote ethnological past. 'Is . . . man . . . under the necessity of making his body a sepulchre for dead carcases, in order to keep himself alive?' is one of Graham's rhetorical questions to which, of course his answer is no. 'The public tables of our steamboats and hotels,' he complains, 'almost literally groan beneath the multitudinous dead that lie in state upon them embalmed and decorated like the bodies of Egyptian potentates emitting their spicy odours to disguise their natural loathsomeness.' But it was to bread that Dr Graham paid the closest attention, and it is in his thinking about this article of diet that he intermingles most intimately facts and faith. In the same paragraph he states, what is undoubtedly true, that when bread forms only a small proportion of a total diet, its exact composition is of minor importance. Then he goes on to assert that 'it is a general and in-variable law of our nature, that all concentrated forms of food are unfriendly to the physiological or vital interests of our bodies . . . nine-tenths of the adults . . . in civil life, are more or less afflicted with obstructions and disturbances in the stomach and bowels . . . and in children and youths, worms, fits, convulsions etc.;' the implica-tion being that they should eat Graham bread made from coarsely ground flour by a method which he particularly describes. And who is to make this bread? 'It is the wife, the mother only, she who loves her husband and her children as a woman ought to love, and who rightly perceives the relations between the dietic habits and physical and moral conditions of her loved ones and justly appreciates the importance of good bread to their physical and moral welfare, she alone it is who will be ever inspired by that cordial and unremitting

[8] Graham, S., *Lectures on the Science of Life*, Boston, 1839.

14

affection and solicitude . . . which are the indispensable attributes of a perfect bread-maker.' It is worth recording that in India today it is an accepted belief that food cooked with love tastes better than food cooked without. And taste is, after all, a valuable part of food.

The magical beliefs about food, as about every other aspect of life, are understandable reactions of men and women living either in a historical period or in a geographical region where scientific knowledge and learning are not available. Such irrational beliefs can be respected almost as a religious faith. Dr Sylvester Graham, with his belief in the virtue of bread made from washed whole grain in love and solicitude, represents a final echo of such irrational faith. For his successors, however, who pick up isolated scientific observations, whose essential usefulness is solely their dependence on reason, and, only half understanding the matters of which they speak, twist them to support some particular perverse non-rational dogma, there can be little sympathy. One of the most misguided of these was W. H. Hay.[9]

Hay seized on two single facts: that the enzyme, ptyalin, present in the mouth is active under alkaline conditions and that the enzyme, pepsin, in the stomach operates under acid conditions. Accepting these as gospel, he abandoned reason and, with the intolerant fervour of a convert, bent all medicine to suit his dogma. First, he asserted, food mainly made up of protein must not be eaten in the same meal as foods which are mainly carbohydrate. From this point, and regardless of the fact that the digestion of protein largely takes place in the acid environment of the stomach, he proceeded to nominate Acid as the arch-fiend of his system of demonology. 'When we eat natural foods in their natural form', he wrote, 'we are not troubled with acid formation, as nature balances these foods very nicely for our digestive ability. But when we introduce the concentrated starches and concentrated proteins we are predisposing ourselves to excessive acid formation.' Then, from asserting that 'life, vitality, health, are synonyms for alkalinity,' he reached the perverse prophetic cry: 'When the causes of disease are understood to be simply an accumulation of the acid end-products of digestion and metabolism in a body unable to eliminate these as fast as they are created, then . . . will the huge mortality . . . sink to almost vanishing point. Then the

[9] Hay, W. H., *A New Health Era*, Harrap, 1935.

expensive diagnostic clinic will fade away . . . and the thing necessary will be an estimation of the extent of accumulation of acid debris.'

The particularly ridiculous feature of this type of teaching is that it bases an intolerant system of unreason on a few selected bits of scientific observation; and science, if it is anything, is the systematization of observed fact to a rational hypothesis. The Hindu eating a diet lacking in beef because he attributes sanctity to cows, and the orthodox Jew prepared to die rather than eat the flesh of pigs, may seem to some misguided, but deserve respect. New-made fallacy built on lack of understanding asks to be corrected.

And all too many fallacies based on ignorant misunderstanding of separate observations have been put about. Stare[10] listed several flagrant examples. In Florida, old people were recommended to consume a daily allocation of sea water. Sea water, it was urged, contains numerous mineral substances in trace amounts, but no consideration was given to whether or not the people who were advised to drink it were in fact suffering from lack of any of these mineral elements. Another common fallacy of the same sort is the contention that fish is good for the brain. To recommend a man to eat an animal's brains to benefit his own is merely to practise the same sort of sympathetic magic that caused the Ashantee chiefs in 1824 to eat the heart of the slain Sir Charles McCarthy,[11] whose courage they admired. But the recommendation of fish arises from ignorance of physiology; the fact that the brain contains a high concentration of phosphorus, as does fish – particularly the bones – does not imply either that the brain becomes deprived of phosphorus when the diet is deficient in it, or that there is any evidence to show that the brains of stupid and forgetful people contain less phosphorus than those of intelligent people with good memories.

The history of medicine contains many instances of sincere physicians who have embraced mistaken ideas. Health is a subtle intermingling of psyche and soma. Generations of eighteenth-century doctors firmly believed that there was sufficient evidence to justify the therapeutic value of blood-letting, just as there were equal numbers of nineteenth-century doctors convinced of the benefits derived from the administration of castor oil. In the twentieth century there was

[10] Stare, F. J., *J. Amer. Geriat. Soc.*, 10, 737, 1962.
[11] Frazer, J. G., *The Golden Bough, Spirits of the Corn and of the Wild*, II, Macmillan, N.Y., 1935.

serious debate as to whether the health of an individual consuming sufficient ascorbic acid to remove any danger of scurvy, say 16 mg. a day, would or would not be improved if his daily intake was raised to, say, 100 mg. such that any more would immediately spill over into his urine. But doubts and debates of this sort are altogether different from fallacies disseminated by interested parties to make money, which must justly be condemned.

Fallacies are of interest to a reflective man only in as much as they make him value the more his own delight in pursuing scientific truth, rather than living either in the dark world of tribal superstition or the even darker world of deception. There is, however, a hazier border-line where food fallacies may be born. This border area is a place where judgement, and often honesty as well, may be clouded by self-interest. It is easy for people learning of the discovery of vitamins, let us say, and of the remarkable effects of a few milligrams of thiamine on a polyneuritic pigeon, or the distressing results on children of a deficiency of vitamin A or vitamin D, to gain a fallacious idea of their power. We have all met people who eat ascorbic acid tablets in the touching belief that they will cure their colds, and thiamine tablets in the certain hope they will ease their rheumatism. These people, though mistaken, can be forgiven for their ignorance. But it is different when a manufacturer advertises that capsules of vitamins A and D cure colds, and that expensive multivitamin tablets protect the well-fed people who can afford them against deficiency diseases they will never experience. Or when the powerful firms marketing confectionery publish to all who will read or listen, that the consumption of sweetmeat A will not make you fat, and that chocolate-bar B is a desirable source of calories—the deliberate implication being that the 'energy' provided by calories is synonymous with 'vigour'.

Dr J. L. Goddard, Commissioner of the US Food and Drugs Administration, has recently drawn attention to the potential harm of fallacies disseminated by manufacturers, even those of the highest standing, who are nevertheless influenced by the insidious pressure of self-interest. First of all, Goddard considered the philosophical question: when the turpitude of an outright quack peddling molasses, let us say, or safflower-seed oil as a panacea for perhaps obesity or heart disease, is compared with that of a respectable firm marketing multivitamin tablets to people among whom the likelihood of vitamin deficiency is remote, to say the least, which way does the moral

17

balance tip?[12] Goddard attacked as fallacies the widely held beliefs that vitamin pills, mineral supplements, dietary preparations and sundry 'health' foods are beneficial to the United States public. In face of this attack, manufacturers protested that their self-interest in the products they market does not blind them to the truth.

But just as there is scope for argument about the exact point at which it is or is not reasonable to agree that claims for 'health' foods and vitamin enrichment are fallacies, so also is there an area of doubt as to the precise level at which it is sensible to assert that the amount of a particular substance in a food is potentially harmful or poisonous. Wholesome food should be clean and free from contamination, yet, just as it is contrary to logic to claim magical virtues for the phosphate content of fish or the brownness of egg-shell or bread, so also may it be unreasonable to cry havoc at the presence of fluorine or arsenic in concentration too low to do harm. It is perhaps an even more perverse fallacy to demand immense precautions against the presence of any trace at all, no matter how little, of, say, an insecticide or weed-killer. It is now recognized that to demand what the United States authorities describe as 'zero tolerance' is a philosophical impossibility. No matter how skilled an analyst may be, he cannot measure nothing.

In 1948, a detailed study was reported[13] of what was called a 'micro-analytical test for purity in food'. The essential features of this analysis were to digest a sample of the foodstuff under test first by boiling it with acid, and then by treating it with the enzyme, pancreatin. The digested mass was then shaken up with a water-immiscible organic solvent which was carefully filtered. Finally, the filter paper was searched with a microscope to see whether any mouse hairs could be found on it. Scientific study had shown that a single small pellet of mouse droppings contains an average of about fifty mouse hairs. The presence of, say, five mouse hairs per pound of biscuits therefore implies that the flour from which they were made had been contaminated by rodents. Does this imply that the biscuits should be rated officially as 'filthy', and condemned? Or is the true implication rather that the flour was made from wheat harvested, not with a combine harvester directly into a sack, but with a reaper and

[12] Anon., *Science*, 152, 1487, 1966.
[13] Kent-Jones, A. J., *et al.*, *Analyst*, 73, 128, 1948.

binder requiring the corn to be stooked to dry in an ecological environment in which field mice have a natural place?

The difficulty of distinguishing wisdom from fallacy when presented with the problem of where to draw the line, has been grotesquely high-lighted by an argument about fish 'flour'.[14][15] This is a product composed of fat-extracted, dried and powdered fish. Incorporated in an impoverished diet, it would contribute protein. The United States Food and Drugs Authority hesitated to approve it as fit for human consumption, not because anybody had ever been harmed by eating it, but because, since it contained the viscera of fish and their contents, as well as fish muscle, it was classified as 'filthy'. By a historical anomaly, whitebait, oysters, clams, cockles and mussels, all of which are offered as human food with their digestive parts in them, are accepted as wholesome.

Science applied to food has achieved much. Knowledge of the chemical components of a nutritious diet has led to the conquest of rickets and such scourges as pellagra, scurvy and beri-beri. Yet chemistry alone is not enough. It is customary for scientists who deal with food facts to refer to fallacies contemptuously and only to denigrate them. Yet they are an aspect of the behaviour of the human species – even that part of it that believes itself to be civilized – which is worthy of study.

[14] Lepper, H. A., *Chem. Eng. News*, 44 (20) 8, 1966.
[15] Campbell, J. W., *Chem. Eng. News,* 44 (25) 7, 1966.

CHAPTER III

MAGIC

'There is no society known,' wrote Mischa Titiev,[1] including our own, that has first made a thorough scientific analysis of all the nutritive elements in its environment and has then given preference to those items that were shown to be best suited to man's bodily needs. Instead, cultural anthropologists find everywhere the existence of food preferences based on symbolic, man-made values that may have nothing to do with nutrition . . .' For example, whereas the Navaho Indians eat gophers as a delicacy, impoverished Caucasoid citizens of the United States refuse them with disgust. And when, in compassion for their poverty, the American Government sent 7-lb. blocks of processed cheese to Karachi, the Pakistanis, taken aback by its alien smell and texture, could find no better use for it than as a raw material for the manufacture of soap. At the same time, mystically convinced of the power of beetles to do harm, American supermarket customers recoil from the presence of these insects in their groceries. It is, therefore, a sign of the enlightenment of American justice to find that these same customers lost their case against the supermarket when the defending lawyer publicly ate a cockroach in court.[2]

Eating is so fundamental an activity that it is understandable that this process, by which alien stuff becomes flesh of a man's flesh, should have remained to the present time entangled in the dark inheritance of magic which clings even to citizens of the scientific age. The magic art is of ancient lineage and wide distribution. It is easy to see that civilization even yet is not entirely devoid of magical belief and ritual. According to J. G. Frazer's definition, magic consists in a pretension by man himself to exert direct control over the forces of nature. Where it is supposed that these forces must be propitiated in order to act favourably towards him, this is religion. Although the world is not so hostile and difficult a place for a modern man to live in as it was for his ignorant savage ancestors, there are yet many

[1] Titiev, M., *The Science of Man*, 2nd ed., Holt, Reinhart & Winston, New York, 1963.
[2] A.P. dispatch in the *Ann Arbor News*, 27 June 1953.

difficulties which remain to be solved and which people may desperately wish to solve.

Deep in the past behind us are the beliefs of our more primitive ancestors who felt themselves to be very directly part of nature and to share the characteristics and virtues of other living things. They felt – and we feel the same when we are happy or sad – that there is a virtue or force which exists, and which some people can to a degree conjure up and command. This force, which was a stuff something like spiritual electricity, was, according to Codrington,[3] called 'mana' by the Melanesians. The same idea has been found to exist among various other peoples, for example, the American Indians, in North Africa and elsewhere. It has come down to us in an explicit form when we compare common water, H_2O, in a dish with the holy water – full of 'mana' powerful to do good – with which a child is baptized. In the Greek ritual of the Dionysiac order, the so-called *omophagia*, or eating of raw flesh, the man is ritually merging himself and his spirit with the virtue of an animal group. And in an entirely different part of the world, the Australian 'kangaroo man' merges his identity with and by his ritual claims strength and kinship with, the kangaroos.[4]

Magic, 'mana', totemism, religion: all these ancient forms are part of the background to modern society and underlie the consciously logical and scientific behaviour by which its members believe they conduct their affairs. Perhaps devout belief in such forces has been lost with the passage of time, although something remains. Nearer to the present scientific age are many of the magical beliefs – things men wished would happen, and thus persuaded themselves they could make to come about – collected by Norman Douglas.[5] The magic here was calculated to give success in love.

Douglas quoted Ovid and Juvenal who described the potency to be derived from eating the 'hippomanes', a fleshy excrescence the size of a fig to be found on the head of a new-born foal. The magical attributes of the mandrake, *Mandragora officinarum*, form a particularly clear example of how such beliefs arise to influence the society that accepts them. They also illustrate the way in which mystical

[3] Codrington, R. H., *The Melanesians*, Oxford, 1891.
[4] Marett, R. R., *Essays presented to C. G. Seligman*, p. 197, ed. Evans-Pritchard, Kegan-Paul, 1934.
[5] Douglas, N., *Paneros: some words on aphrodisiacs and the like*, Chatto & Windus, 1931.

21

faith and measurable biochemical fact may become merged and intermingled.

The mandrake is a plant of the Solanaccae family to which the potato also belongs. It is a native of the Mediterranean area. The plant has a short stem bearing a tuft of purple, bell-like flowers which subsequently yield orange-coloured berries. These berries ripen in May and can grow to the size of small apples. The Arabs call them Devil's Apples and find their smell enticing. Reference to this attractive smell is made in the Song of Solomon.[6] The root is thick, fleshy and often forked. Seeing this divided root, the people of ancient times were reminded of the two legs of a man, and, before long – by the customary reasoning of sympathetic magic – they claimed for it the powers of a love philtre. And because the plant was believed to possess such powers, it needed only a little more faith to claim that there was evidence – as there was once for angels with wings, and is now for space saucers and UFOs – that the plant shrieked when it was touched. 'And shrieks like mandrakes torn out of the earth, that living mortals, hearing them, run mad,' wrote Shakespeare in *Romeo and Juliet*. A twentieth-century citizen may no longer believe this, but belief in the Book of Genesis is not long past; and there[7] the faith in the mandrake's power to aggravate concupiscence is explicitly accepted. 'And Reuben went in the days of the wheat harvest, and found mandrakes in the field and brought them to his mother Leah. Then Rachel said to Leah, Give me, I pray thee, of thy son's mandrakes. And she said unto her, Is it a small matter that thou hast taken my husband? and wouldst thou take away my son's mandrakes also? And Rachel said, Therefore he shall lie with thee tonight for thy son's mandrakes.'

A modern scholar who wishes also to be, so far as is possible, that legal paragon 'a reasonable man', needs to know and understand the old magical beliefs attached to different foods, if he hopes success-fully to influence the diet of a community. But it is not enough to classify beliefs black or white, that is to say, scientifically true on the one hand and superstitious error on the other. The perverse logic of the 'Doctrine of Signatures', which lies at the very heart of primitive magic, is clearly nonsense. The juice of red beet is *not* of particular value to anaemic women, because blood is red too, as the Doctrine

[6] Song of Solomon, VII, 13.
[7] Genesis, XXX, 14–16.

22

would insist; neither is the yellow celandine a cure for yellow jaundice, although this is widely believed among credulous people. It is, therefore, equally ridiculous to suppose that mandrake stimulates the sexual powers simply because its root bears some resemblance to a man's crotch. Unluckily, however, for those who hold to the rational, demonstrable truths of logic, the matter, as so often happens in nature, is not entirely clear-cut and definite. The shape of the mandrake's root has, indeed, no bearing on its physiological effect. But the fact that it does exert an effect is well established. In Africa and the East it is used here and there as a narcotic and anti-spasmodic, and in ancient times, according to Isidorus and Serapion, it was eaten to diminish sensitivity to pain and thus help patients to endure surgical operations. Shakespeare again refers to its narcotic powers when he causes Cleopatra to say: 'Give me to drink mandragora . . . That I might sleep out this great gap of time My Antony away.'[8] And in *Othello*[9] we find the passage 'Not poppy, nor mandragora, Nor all the drowsy syrops of the world, Shall ever medicine thee to that sweet sleep Which thou ow'dst yesterday'.

The conclusion emerges from these facts that, while the superstitious magical belief in the reason for using mandrake as a love-potion had no more truth and virtue in ancient times than has the modern belief that laxatives produce 'inner cleanliness' and must therefore be beneficial, yet the scholar must at the same time appreciate that mandrake does contain pharmacologically-active compounds which might steady the nerves and hence improve the performance of a timid lover.

This is but a single example of the way in which ancient magical nonsense may have mixed with it odd nuggets of truth. Perhaps, therefore, Douglas was not entirely wasting his time in writing, nor are we necessarily wasting ours in reading the beliefs of the Arabs that the use of 'brazed relics of the skink' – a desert animal – excites the procreative faculties, that consumption of asparagus or leeks improves amative performance, as the Doctrine of Signatures would obviously suggest, and that a parallel belief (also in harmony with the same doctrine) is that love is strengthened in a man or woman who eats turtle-doves or partridges. But the way in which magical beliefs, in themselves irrational superstition, may lead to real and solid

[8] Antony and Cleopatra, I, v, 4.
[9] Othello, II, iii, 331.

progress is shown by the history of the magical Doctrine of Signatures itself.

The origin of the Doctrine dates from primitive antiquity. It took shape as a definite philosophy, however, in the sixteenth century when Parcelsus gathered together the agglomeration of primitive ideas into some sort of coherent form. Its principles were, firstly, that like cures like, that is, that red beet 'makes' blood (as the ancients believed) or, as twentieth-century ladies in British public houses assert, dark red port is a 'tonic' wine. The second principle of the Doctrine of Signatures was that everything in nature, animal, plant or vegetable, always carried with it the characteristics of its own appearance and properties. Added to this was the very ancient belief that man, and the world and all the things in it, bore to each other the relationship of microcosm to macrocosm. This meant that man in little reflected the properties of everything in the big world of his environment. And Paracelsus, who was a mystic and a believer in astrology, born Theophrastus von Holenheim in 1493 near the southern end of the Lake of Zürich, codified the beliefs which together made up the Doctrine. But he did more than this. He extended the Doctrine by a further principle which asserted that all bodies contained in varying proportion sulphur, which induced change, combustibility, volatilization and growth; salt which provided stability and non-inflammability; and, finally, mercury which gave fluidity.[10]

However obscure, his symbolic language did contain a seed of truth, out of which solid progress grew. For, in formulating a thesis that the properties of a food could be measured in terms of its chemical composition, he was pointing the way to the science of nutrition which, four centuries later, was built on this same principle. At the same time, Paracelsus began the overthrow of the Galenic system which prescribed mixtures of heterogeneous herbs and odd fragments of animals, not excluding their excrement.

Man is slow to learn. And human behaviour is difficult to influence. The twentieth-century 'health' food shops remain as monuments to the mysticism of antiquity in an allegedly scientific society carrying on the magical Doctrine of Signatures passed by Paracelsus to Giamballesta Porta whose book, *Phytognomonica*, was published in

[10] Arber, A., *Herbals*, Cambridge U.P., 1938.

24

Naples in 1588.[11] In it he asserted that by eating long-lived plants a man would lengthen his life, while by eating short-lived ones he would shorten it. Herbs with yellow sap healed jaundice, those with rough outer surfaces healed diseases that make the skin rough. Plants thought to resemble butterflies cured insect bites, those with angular-jointed parts were remedies for the stings of scorpions. Current credulity on remedies for baldness give twentieth-century readers no right to scoff at pre-scientific faith in the consumption of the maidenhair, a plant with fine leaf stalks, as a veritable cure for this condition. And so on.

In England, the Doctrine flourished in the works of Nicholas Culpeper and William Coles, who wrote a book called *Adam in Eden*. Radcliff Salaman[12] quotes Coles as claiming: 'The Wallnut is a cure for troubles of the brain.' The reasoning for this belief, of course, was that the outer fleshy husk of a walnut was taken to represent the scalp, the shell the bony skull, and the inner, convoluted kernel resembled the shape of the lobes of the brain.

The narrative traced by Salaman of the entanglement of the potato with the confused strands of magic which are so much a part of the irrational aspect of human thinking, exemplifies very well the factors of which an informed nutritionist must be aware if he pretends to understand his subject. The potato first appeared in Europe at the end of the sixteenth century. It was the first edible plant to be grown from tubers and not from seed. No other known food possessed underground stems on which there grew white or flesh-coloured nodules. The entire appearance and behaviour of the plant were strange and it excited interest, suspicion and fear. The immediate questions were: what 'signature' did it bear? what warning did it convey? Strange foods to this day are treated with suspicion. To European farmers of the seventeenth century, the white nodular tubers with their bulbous, finger-like growths, recalled the deformed hands and bleached skin of leprosy, the dreaded disease of the Middle Ages and the Renaissance.

The irrationality of magic makes it impossible to forecast the responses of its devotees. Paracelsus' Doctrine of Signatures allows both red beet, *unlike* the paleness of a sufferer from anaemia, to cure

---

[11] Arber, A., *Herbals*, Cambridge U.P., 1938.
[12] Salaman, R., *The History and Social Influence of the Potato*, Cambridge U.P., 1949.

his complaint and make his blood redder – which, of course, it does not do; or the yellow celandine, *like* the yellow complexion of the patient with jaundice, to cure it. Which way would the thinking, if as such it can be described, about the new and unfamiliar potato go? Paracelsus himself, likening the date to a cancerous tumour, claimed it to be a specific cure. His successors, however, recognizing the signature of leprosy in the potato, condemmned it as the cause. The opposition to its use was widespread throughout Europe. How it was overcome, if this can be learned, provides a lesson for modern food scientists.

At first the prejudice fixed on leprosy. When this could no longer be used for blame, the disease having dwindled, scrofula was used as an excuse. 'The scrofulous are common in Switzerland,' wrote Daniel Langhaus, a Swiss physician in 1768,[13] 'where the people support themselves above all on potatoes. I am persuaded, myself, that the scrofulous troubles which prevail in our Cantons are entirely the result of this harmful dietary and the lack of exercise. The proof of which is that they are extremely rare in countries where the potato is unknown.'

Man, the thinking animal *par excellence*, is indeed his own worst enemy. And in the dogged persistence with which he clings to non-sensical and pernicious magic, shows remarkable pertinacity in his twisted will to harm himself. Having first discarded the pretext that the potato was a cause of leprosy, he next gave up the belief in its malevolent magic power to produce scrofula, but then complained that it caused 'fever' – which may have been typhoid, typhus or half a dozen other infectious diseases then of unknown origin. This accusation was particularly prevalent in France up to the nineteenth century. There, famines in the south had produced epidemics which were attributed to the one thing – the potato – which in fact had prevented absolute disaster, and which, but for the prejudice derived from its unfavourable magical 'signature', might have prevented famine altogether.[14]

To understand magic and know what it does is one thing, to overcome it, even in an age of enlightenment, is another. In Prussia in the

[13] Quoted by Roze, E., *Histoire de la Pomme de Terre*, Rothschild, Paris, 1898.
[14] Salaman, R., *The History and Social Influence of the Potato*, Cambridge U.P., 1949.

26

eighteenth century, people believed that potatoes gave rise not only to scrofula, but to consumption, rickets and other diseases as well. See how subtly the black of the old magic had become intertwined with the white of the new scientific knowledge that was to come. Potatoes do not *cause* tuberculosis – that is, consumption – or rickets, any more than they cause scrofula. Nevertheless, people living under impoverished conditions, in poor housing, and eating an inadequate diet of which potato could very well form a major component, *would* be susceptible to tuberculosis infection; and their young children, if their diet or that of their mothers before the infants were born, lacked milk and butter, fish, eggs or other sources of vitamin D, could also be expected to contract rickets. This does not imply that magic is credible, rather it reinforces the importance of a rational attack on it.

Frederick the Great in 1774 set out to attack magic. He sent a wagon-load of potatoes to Kolberg, following a period of acute scarcity, in the hope that the people there would appreciate their usefulness and start growing them for themselves. But the citizens merely sent a message back saying: 'The things have neither smell nor taste, not even dogs will eat them, so what use are they to us?'[15] In the end, the Emperor was compelled to dispatch a Swabian gendarme who eventually succeeded, partly by eating potatoes himself and partly by persuasion, in getting the peasants to use them. The French authorities encountered the same difficulties. As late as 1771, as in Germany, the population were still deeply suspicious of potatoes, and without reason, only echoing without knowing they were doing so their fear of their bad magical properties. In this instance the Government took the direct scientific approach, and invited the Medical Faculty of Paris to undertake an inquiry. Their verdict was that the potato was a good and healthy food, in no way injurious to health, and of great utility.[16] In the 1777 edition of *La Grande Encyclopédie*, the distinguished agricultural scientist, Samuel Engel, used (to combat popular belief in its unwholesomeness) the argument that in Ireland, where potatoes were by then the staple food, the peasants were not only strong and vigorous, but particularly liable to beget twins.

It is interesting to compare the ways in which the men of the eighteenth-century Enlightenment attempted to understand and

[15] Bruford, W. H., *Germany in the Eighteenth Century*, Cambridge U.P., 1935.
[16] Arber, A., *Herbals*, Cambridge U.P., 1938.

hence move forwards from the obscurity of pre-scientific thinking, with the approach of twentieth-century nutritionists to the same problem. In 1940, a number of Western-trained scientists set about improving the diet of a community of Zulus living in a 'native reserve' in South Africa.[17] That there was need for improvement was shown by the crude mortality rate of 38 per 1,000 of the population, and the infant mortality rate of 276 per 1,000 live births – that is to say, 276 infants out of each 1,000 born died before their first birthday. In addition to this, many of the people showed signs of ill-health directly attributable to malnutrition. Two diseases – pellagra, due to insufficiency of the vitamin niacin, and kwashiorkor, due to inadequate protein – occurred among them.

The scientists carried out a dietary survey and found that in one special group of mothers and children the principal article of food was maize, cooked and prepared in a number of different ways, and only sometimes supplemented with dried beans, trifling amounts of milk, and, very occasionally, some meat and greens. When the season was right they ate potatoes and pumpkins, but they drank large quantities of millet beer all the year round. This diet, based on their own African culture, was affected by the culture of the wealthy and technological West only when absent members of the community, seeking their fortunes as labourers in the gold mines and factories of South Africa, sent home as gifts parcels of 'refined' maize meal, and money, with which the women bought sugar and white bread.

This was the diet of the mothers whose children died before a twelvemonth or survived to develop kwashiorkor.

But when the Western scientists attempted to explain that the cause of the ill-health and death was an inadequate diet, and went on to give lectures about proteins and vitamins, calling them 'body-building' and 'protective' agents measured in grams and milligrams, the people failed to understand. The material philosophy of the West was too remote from the spiritual philosophy of Africa. The babies died and the children sickened because of diverse gods and spirits and forces. Had not their ancestors, asked the Zulu women, always eaten as they ate, and yet they were strong and powerful people?

Dr John Cassel, the man in charge of the work, and his colleagues, had the wisdom to see that the doctrine of science, although eagerly

[17] Cassel, J., *Amer. J. Pub. Health*, 47, 732, 1957.

embraced by the girl students of London and Glasgow, Boston and Amsterdam, was not converting the mothers in whose midst the Pholela Health Centre had been set up. They shifted their ground, therefore, and began to expound, not the alien science, but the history of the Zulus themselves. Having searched the records, they found that, far from its being their traditional food, maize meal had only been introduced into the dietary of the Zulus and other Bantu-speaking tribes by white settlers. Before their arrival, the people used millet as their main cereal. But, more important than this, they had been a roving pastoral nation possessing large herds of cattle, and eating meat. Milk had also been an important ingredient of their diet; no meal had been thought complete unless milk had been drunk with it. At that time, the land provided wild game, roots, berries and green vegetables as well.

As soon as the Western teachers obtained confirmation of these facts from old men and women who remembered these things, they began to win credence for other items of their doctrine as well; for example, that unborn infants might perhaps be influenced by the diet of their mothers, and that the sole purpose of food might be more than just to fill the belly, that one food might make a man strong while another might make him fat. To teach that foods were composed of nutrients – substances of a specific chemical composition which exerted specific physiological effects – presented a more serious problem. For example, the women drank no milk and were not interested in talk of its content of protein, vitamins and calcium. No one, man, woman or child, would drink milk from a cow belonging to a family other than their own. To do so would be contrary to nature and decency and would bring inevitable evil on their heads. Women, least of all, could drink milk. Had they not themselves come as brides from an outside family? Furthermore, it was accepted belief that women during their menses or when pregnant exerted an evil influence on cattle. They were, as a consequent matter of normal prudence, never allowed either to pass near the cattle enclosures or to drink milk. Only under two conditions might a married woman drink milk: if her father gave her her own cow as a wedding present she could safely milk it for her own use, or if her husband slaughtered a goat with appropriate ceremony. Unfortunately, the poverty of the community was such that the possibility of carrying out either of these exercises had become rare.

The origin for this taboo against women drinking milk was obscure. It appeared to be based on the belief in the links between a man, his cattle and his ancestors. The bonds of magic are stronger than the bonds of reason. A Zulu would no sooner drink milk from his neighbour's cow even if he were starving, than a Yorkshireman would, albeit in the last extremity of want, eat his neighbour's amputated leg, although this Western taboo does not inhibit his accepting his neighbour's kidney should the neighbour be prepared to offer it as a graft.

When Dr Cassel and his colleagues understood why the Bantu people failed to accept the argument that milk was a vehicle for protein and vitamins, and appreciated that to them milk was indissolubly linked to the particular cow from which it came (this cow being an integral part of the family to which it belonged), then it was possible to do something sensible about it. Since it was not acceptable to drink milk belonging to a particular family or tribe with which one was personally acquainted – rather in the same way that some Western people feel a conscience-stricken revulsion against eating a pet rabbit with whom they have been on terms of long-continued friendship – what could be simpler than to introduce 'detribalized' milk? Supplies of powdered milk were introduced. Even though no secret was made of the fact that the basis from which it had been manufactured had been derived from a cow, the most orthodox of mothers-in-law and husbands had no objection to its being used by the young women of their tribe. The moral link had been broken. And in any event, the original cows had never belonged to Bantu people. Eventually, having got used to drinking reconstituted dried milk, the more 'modern' and educated women began to drink the milk of their family cows.

After twelve years' work and persuasion, when milk of one sort or another was a part of the diet of some of the women and some of the children, when some of the families had gardens and all of them had advice, the infant mortality rate dropped from 276 to 96, pellagra and kwashiorkor had become rare, and the average weight of one-year-old babies was two pounds greater than it had been before. This was progress, but progress due as much to the understanding of human behaviour as to the understanding of science. An anonymous contributor to the *Lancet*,[18] writing in 1967, pointed out the universality of

[18] Anon., *Lancet*, I, vol. I, 674, 1967.

the belief of Rhodesian Africans in magic and witchcraft. Almost everyone is quite convinced that a *muroyi*, or hereditary witch, can bewitch a victim by entering his hut at night and merely touching him. Other kinds of witches are able to bewitch the meat or beer of those against whom they work their magic.

The Africans accept the witch and his magic as part of life, just as the European and North American accept the existence of toxic contaminants of food or the pathogenic bacteria by which they are surrounded, not knowing who will be struck down by disease or food poisoning. In Western communities there is fear of falling a victim to typhoid from contaminated corned beef in Aberdeen, to becoming a statistic in the incidence of coronary heart disease from eating too much fat or sugar, or to being laid low by gastritis while holiday-making in North Africa. The mob may vindictively pursue a food manufacturer, a cook, a medical officer of health, or the Government – sometimes with as little justification as is shown by an African widower when, in fact, the laws of probability are all that are involved. The African behaviour may, sometimes – but not always – constitute a simplified model by which Western prejudice and hysteria can be assessed. The Western approach to magic can only justly claim superiority, where reason has been used to assess the facts. Acceptance of scientists as all-wise and all-powerful is little short of a witch-doctor cult.

A different aspect of the magic attached to eating and drinking is derived from the fact that many races are convinced that when a man eats or drinks his soul may escape through his mouth and, to avoid this and prevent their enemies gaining an advantage over them at this time, the members of such races carefully cover their faces when they eat or turn away and take their meals in secret.[19] Who can say that the modern Western custom by which employers and people who consider themselves to be of the superior classes take care to eat separately from those whom they employ, or those they think are their inferiors, may not be derived from the same distant root?

According to Malinowski,[20] there are two fundamental principles on which magic is based. One of them is to blame a human being for

[19] Frazer, J. G., *The Golden Bough, Taboos and the Perils of the Soul*, Macmillan, 1935.

[20] Malinowski, B., *The Dynamics of Culture Change*, ed. Kaberry, P. M., Yale U.P., 1945.

misfortune, and thus reduce the metaphysical and fatalistic elements in one's reaction to it. An African mother, by blaming a jealous neighbour for putting a spell on her child's food, can ease her grief at its death. A civilized person can blame food manufacturers or government regulations enforcing the fluoridization of drinking water or the vitaminization of margarine, for all the ill-health of the community. There is more hope in counteracting human machinations than in dealing with the decrees of fate or the will of God. From this point of view, although belief in magic is nonsense, it can be seen to possess a comprehensible psychological basis. Furthermore, belief in magic may not always be an unmitigated evil; it may be a source at least of comfort and hope, a handle to manage the unmanageable. A clear-headed attempt to free a population from the incubus of magic may therefore deprive them of something more than their superstitions.

The second principle of magic identified by Malinowski is an extension of the first. Just as an individual African may lay the blame on his enemy for having put a spell on his food, or as a European may lay the blame for nervous prostration, generalized malaise or incapacitating migraine on margarine or sardines (yet suffer no ill from a dish in which, unknown to him, these articles are present as ingredients), so too may social groups blame whole categories of people for laying harmful spells upon them. Since witchcraft is based on scapegoat psychology, the most likely people to be blamed are those with whom conflict most readily occurs. Malinowski goes further when he writes: 'The common measure between the rational and logical approach to witchcraft and belief [in it] must be looked for in the sociological context of human malice, competition and sense of injury which form the actual framework in social relationships upon which the supernatural power has always to work.' The general belief in malevolent witchcraft in Africa and remote parts of the world, in South America and Oceania, is paralleled in its most pernicious form by the pursuit of spies in Great Britain in World War I, the mindless attacks on 'saboteurs' and 'Trotskyists' in Russia, and – most monstrous of all – the insane slaughter of the Jews in Germany. There spills over from this some splashes of magic in the pejorative identification of foreigners with unfamiliar foods. This makes the French frogs, the Germans krauts and the English limies.

It is sound scientific knowledge, that is to say 'the truth' – and some people might say 'the whole truth' – that nutritional wellbeing and health are due to the consumption of food providing appropriate amounts of calories, of protein in adequate quantity, and of the correct amino acid composition, the necessary minerals and those vitamins found by trial and experiment to be required for the proper functioning of human metabolic processes. This being so, we must condemn those people who believe that they 'cannot eat' sardines or that they will be prostrated by margarine. But although the truth of nutritional science is surely based, and – though it may be modified and extended – cannot be overthrown, there is a limit to its applicability. Perfect nutrition is, by definition one must conclude, what will produce health. It is the difficulty or defining health that is the weak point in the definition of good nutrition.

Dr Johnson's dictionary says that 'health is the state of being hale, sound or whole, or freedom from sickness, pain or disease'. Or that it is, 'welfare of mind, moral wellbeing, a state of salvation, purity, goodness or Divine Grace'.[21] Nearly two hundred years later, the World Health Organization in their definition remained closer to Dr Johnson than might have been expected when, at a meeting in June 1946, they defined health as 'a state of complete physical, mental and social wellbeing and not merely the absence of disease or infirmity'.[22] This state must clearly depend on something more than a supply of necessary foodstuffs, even supplemented by shelter and clothing and the absence of pathogenic micro-organisms. The introduction of the idea of social wellbeing may also involve magic which is very much an attribute of society.

That death may be brought about by magic, exorcism and the casting of spells is well established.[23] And although it can be argued that magic is nonsense, the measurable physiological effects brought about by the psychological condition of a bewitched victim are every bit as real as those due to anorexia or hypoglycaemia. Unquestionably death is the ultimate antithesis of health which it is the object of the nutritionist to promote. A normal man is in intimate relationship with his environment upon which his wellbeing depends. When he feels hunger, it can be argued that the mechanism at work is triggered off by a critical drop in the concentration of glucose in his circulating

Johnson, S., *Dictionary*, London, 1755.
WHO, International Health Conference, New York, 1946.
Cannon, W. B., 'Voodoo Death', *Amer. Anthropol.*, XLIV, 1942.

bloodstream. But the human circumstance is more complex than this. Not only must the subtle organization of a man with his family and neighbours (by means of which food is produced, prepared and served at appropriate times, and in the form of acceptable meals) be in good working order, but in most societies – and particularly in those of the industrialized West – the even more complicated economic system by which money is distributed must also exist. During the 1930s, there were gluts of unsold food in America while men of the same cultural group suffered from want elsewhere. The effect was as if a magic spell fixed men's limbs immovable so that both the ruined producers of food in the countryside, and the hungry townspeople, stood helplessly by unable to do what all of them recognized to be sensible.

When a sorcerer casts a voodoo spell over a man, and his neighbours know that this has been done, the victim of the sorcery, according to Cannon,[24] is thoroughly convinced that he is doomed. His friends and relatives share this certainty, and the community of which he is a member treats him as if he were already dead. Torn from all his family and social ties, and excluded from all functions and activities through which he experienced self-awareness, the victim of magic becomes cut off from the multiple reference system by which a normal individual lives. In our own society, an old bachelor living alone may suffer, or even die, from malnutrition. Not because he lacks money to buy food, or is ignorant of his needs, but just because 'it does not seem worth while to cook just for myself'. There is, indeed, a well-known clinical state recognized as 'bachelor scurvy' arising from this very cause.

Lévi-Strauss[25] has described the situation thus: 'There is . . . no reason to doubt the efficiency of certain magic practices. But at the same time we see that the efficiency of magic implies a belief in magic. The latter has three complementary aspects: first, the sorcerer's belief in the effectiveness of his techniques; second, the patient's or victim's belief in the sorcerer's power; and, finally, the faith and expectations of the group, which constantly act as a sort of gravitational field within which the relationship between sorcerer and bewitched is located and defined.'

[24] Malinowski, B., *The Dynamics of Culture Change*, ed. Kaberry, P. M., Yale U.P., 1945.
[25] Lévi-Strauss, C., *Structural Anthropology*, Basic Books, New York, 1963.

The dissolution of his social personality has a direct effect on the physical integrity of the man upon whom the magic spell is laid. Hopelessness and particularly fear, like rage, affect the sympathetic nervous system. Under normal circumstances, the physiological response is useful, allowing the individual to adapt himself to the new situation. But when the customary social frame of reference is withdrawn, as it is when the victim is known to have been put under a magic spell, the sympathetic nervous system produces a disorganized and intensified response. This can lead within a few hours to a decrease in blood volume with a consequent drop in blood pressure. This results in damage to the circulatory system which may be permanent or fatal. The decrease in blood volume is accentuated by the growing permeability of the capillary vessels. The nutritional response is a rejection of food and drink which contributes still further to the crisis.

Lévi-Strauss has drawn attention to a remarkable report published in the London *Sunday Times* of 22 April 1956. An Australian aborigine was brought into the hospital in Darwin apparently dying of sorcery. He was placed in an oxygen tent and fed intravenously. Two things happened. The treatment he received, to be sure, prevented any further deterioration of his physical condition, but – and this was of more permanent benefit – the sight of the Western ju-ju men and women, purposefully moving about in their ritual robes of white, some with the lower parts of their faces concealed, others bringing mysterious objects, bottles of blood, wheeled carts carrying great iron cylinders and pulsating bellows, while the man himself was hooded in a transparent cover, convinced him that white man's magic was the stronger.

Taken by itself, the mechanism of magic can be seen to be false. Except by accident, the Doctrine of Signatures does not stand up to examination. There will have been men who ate walnuts yet whose brain-power remained palpably negligible, just as good observers will have seen their neighbours to be cowards in spite of their diet of lions' hearts. And just as magic and its mumbo-jumbo can be seen to be false, nutritional science, taken by itself, can be demonstrated by experimental fact to be true. But it is only true for isolated tissue cultures in test-tubes or rats in cages. During World War II, the British Red Cross Society applied all the resources of science to insure that the composition of the parcels sent to prisoners of war was such that they contained all the nutrients necessary for nutritional health. And they did indeed save their recipients from malnutrition and the diseases of vitamin deficiency. Yet the cruellest punishment their jailers could mete out was, not to deprive the prisoners of them, but, after having opened them in their presence and displayed the chocolate, the meat loaf, the biscuits and the dried milk, to pound the whole lot to a mush. The nourishment remained, but the sight of the broken mess could reduce a man to a state of hysterical despair.

Before he jeers at the African dying from the magic spell laid upon him by the tribal sorcerer, and at the relatives and friends who withdraw from the victim in resignation as if he were already dead, the Western citizen, strong in his faith in the truth and power of science, should consider his erstwhile business colleague. This was a man, healthy and prosperous before, busy in his office, happy in his secretary and his subordinates, lunching regally with his equals whom he addressed by their first names and who did the same to him, playing golf and drinking drinks. Then the day came and the spell was cast. Ritual speeches were spoken and ritual tokens presented – a clock, an armchair, a motor-mower – and the victim was declared 'retired'. His old colleagues withdrew, there were no longer any lunches, secretaries or business contacts. No physical harm was done to the victim, he still had enough to eat, shelter, clothing and warmth. But his frame of reference was broken, the social context in which he had previously lived was destroyed and, like the African victim of sorcery, the 'magic' might soon prove fatal and he would die.

CHAPTER IV

THE COMPULSION OF CUSTOM

The fact remains that men and women living in the societies which make up the human population do not ingest nutrients, they consume foods. More than this, they eat meals. Although to the single-minded biochemist or physiologist, this aspect of human behaviour may appear to be irrelevant or even frivolous, it is nevertheless a deeply ingrained part of the human situation which exerts a very direct and profound effect on nutritional status and health.

Community habits and customs may benefit health and physiological wellbeing, or they may harm them. And a scientist or sociologist investigating any particular situation needs to take a clear look and exercise calm judgement before reaching a conclusion. In few areas of human behaviour do the early conditioning of customary use and inbred tradition exert so subtle an effect on the mind, not only of the people being studied but of the scientific investigator as well. Few Englishwomen, trained to use all their intellectual facilities at Oxford University, stop to question the truth of what they assert with such authority to their husbands and children, that a *hot* breakfast of porridge, bacon and eggs is essential for proper nutrition regardless of the evidence of the millions outside England who subsist without these items in the morning. And few equally well-educated Americans would challenge the allegedly scientific basis of the importance for optimal human efficiency of a daily glass of orange-juice.

In 1945 a study[1] was made of the state of nutrition of the Otomi Indians in the Mezquital Valley in Mexico. The health of these people was found to be good, yet they were eating few of the foods usually considered in the Western world to be necessary for a nutritious diet. They ate little meat, dairy produce, fruit or vegetables of conventional kinds. Instead they made their meals from tortillas and from local plants such as malva, hediondilla, tuna, nopales, maguey, garambullo, yucca, purslane, pigweed, sorrel, wild mustard flowers, *lengua de vaca*, sow-thistle and cactus fruit. They drank pulque, an intoxicating beverage made from the juice of the century

[1] Anderson, R. K., and Calvo, J., *et al., Amer. J. Pub. Health*, 36, 883, 1946.

plant. Yet when the components of the Otomi Indians' diet were
flown to the Massachusetts Institute of Technology and analysed,[2]
it was found that they provided a better nutritional balance than was
present in the diet of a group of United States town-dwellers surveyed not long before.[3]

Sir Robert McCarrison in the early decades of this century was
seized with the importance of the choice of diet by different races in
India. 'Nothing could be more striking,' he wrote,[4] 'than the contrast
between the manly, stalwart and resolute races of the north – the
Pathans, Baluchis, Sikhs, Punjabis, Rajputs and Maharattas – and
the poorly-developed, toneless and supine people of the east and
south; Bengalis, Madrassis, Kanarese and Travancorians . . . Inherited factors, climate, customs, caste, religion and endemic diseases
no doubt contribute their share to the production of this result; but
food is the paramount factor concerned. This is shown to be so by an
experiment carried out . . . in this laboratory.[5] Groups of young rats –
twenty in each – were fed on certain national diets of India; care
being taken to simulate in every detail the culinary practices of the
races concerned. The experiment was so conducted that factors such
as climate, atmospheric temperature, rainfall, age, body-weight, sex-
distribution, caging, housing and hygiene were the same in all
groups.' And then he went on to detail the results of the experiment,
how the average weight of the animals fed on the Sikh diet of freshly-
ground whole wheat made into cakes of unleavened bread, milk,
butter, ghee, curds, legumes, fresh carrots, cabbage and other
vegetables, and meat once a week, was 235 grams at the end of the
trial while, on the other hand, the group of rats fed on the Madrassi
diet weighed only 155 grams. Their diet was composed of washed
polished rice, legumes, condiments, vegetable oil, coffee with sugar
and a little milk, ghee used sparingly, and coconut.

Here we have an example, as McCarrison described it, of two
groups of Indians eating different diets. What they ate differed partly
because of the difference in the supplies of food available in the
districts in which they lived, but the difference was also due, as he
stated, to 'inherited factors, customs, caste and religion'. An equally

[2] Gravioto, B. R., *et al.*, *J. Nutrition*, 23, 317, 1945.
[3] Lockhart, E. E., *et al.*, *J. Amer. Dietet. Ass.*, 20, 742, 1944.
[4] McCarrison, R., *Indian J. Med. Res.*, 19, 61, 1931.
[5] McCarrison, R., *Brit. Med. J.*, ii, 730, 1926.

striking difference was described by two equally distinguished scientists, Orr and Gilks – Dr Orr later on became Lord Boyd Orr, first director general of the Food and Agriculture Organization of the United Nations. These two men studied the food eaten by two nations, the Kikuyu and the Masai, in Africa.[6] The Kikuyu were found to be settled, agricultural people living on a mainly vegetarian diet. This was largely composed of cereals, tubers, legumes, plantains and green vegetables. Their neighbours, the Masai, were a pastoral community. They ate maize, bananas, beans and cereals, to be sure, but in addition they consumed the products of their cattle, partly in the form of milk, as is common in the West, and partly in the form of blood, which they drew from time to time for their own sustenance without harming the beasts. As I have commented before, it is curious that Western nations accept into their system blood from only one species of living animal – man. Of course, the Masai also ate the flesh of their cattle when the time did come to terminate their lives.

The remarkable divergences between the diets selected by the Kikuyu and the Masai were reflected, as might have been expected, in their physiological state. The Kikuyu, on their predominantly carbohydrate diet, were observed by Orr and Gilks to be lethargic, lacking in stamina and subject to disease. The Masai were on average five inches taller, twenty-three pounds heavier, and had 50 per cent greater muscular strength. Bone defects, dental decay, anaemia, ulcers and bronchitis were more common among the Kikuyu than the Masai. For instance, 63 per cent of the Kikuyu boys had bone deformities, 40 per cent had decayed teeth, 48 per cent of them had anaemia, and 33 per cent of them suffered from ulcers of one sort or another. The comparable figures for Masai boys were 12, 8, 12 and 3 per cent. Not all the sufferings of the Kikuyu were due to their choice of diet, but Orr and Gilks attributed much of their inferiority to the Masai to what they ate.

Two American scientists, Furnas and Furnas[7], have asserted that the races of mankind, left to themselves, will eat almost everything available, so that the contents of their stomachs tend to contain a cross-section of the edible fauna and flora of the region they inhabit. This is not strictly accurate. As we have already seen, the mechanistic

[6] Orr, J. G., and Gilks, J. L., Med. Res. Council, *Spec. Rep. Ser.*, 155, 1931.
[7] Furnas, C. C., and Furnas, S. M., *Man, Bread and Destiny*, Cassell, London, 1938.

image of man as a biochemical engine, for which all metabolizable foodstuffs serve as grist to the mill, is an inaccurate overstatement. The observations of McCarrison and of Orr and Gilks alone, demonstrate the inadequacy of this idea. At the same time, habits and customs can only operate upon what is available.

It is a striking feature of dietetic history that, as the centuries have passed and human life has become more complex and sophisticated, the number of different edible foods which are actually eaten has steadily dwindled. Modern man has reduced himself to a diet made up of a very few species of cereals, tubers, fruits and vegetables, and the products derived from a limited number of domesticated animals. This is only partly due to the fact that it is most economical to process large quantities of a single, uniform product. The yield per acre of standardized, inbred wheat in Canada is not very great, but it is convenient to be able to harvest large areas of it with big machines, extract white flour in enormous mills, and convert it into uniform loaves of bread in equally large and highly-automated bakeries. Yet this is only one of the reasons for the limited standardized diet of twentieth-century people. Early in the century, whales were slaughtered in large numbers. Their meat, one could have assumed, would have been well-suited to become a staple article of diet. It is reasonable to assume that part of it at least could have been processed and distributed. Yet, while it is eaten by more primitive societies, the more socially advanced nations showed little interest in it, and the largest animals on earth were exterminated principally to allow margarine – a foodstuff that *is* accepted by nations of the technological group – to be manufactured. The selection of one substance as an article of diet rather than another is clearly influenced as much by the conscious choice of the tribe as by availability.

Why different groups of people choose their food differently is an interesting problem to which there is so far no clear and absolute answer. There are, however, a number of general factors to explain how differences in food habits came about and what it is that causes communities to hold on to them with the fixity they do. Consider the use of insects for food.

Under normal circumstances, the average white inhabitants of Europe and America will refuse with disgust any offer of insects for culinary purposes. According to Bodenheimer,[8] this conspicuous

[8] Bodenheimer, F. S., *Insects as Human Food*, Junk, The Hague, 1951.

aversion is a prejudice acquired incidentally to the progress of civiliz-ation. It falls into the same category as the prejudice against raw meat and raw fish, and against eating frogs, oysters, crayfish and *frutti di mare* held by those European communities which happen to be unfamiliar with them. The prejudice, a purely emotional influence fixed in the minds of 'advanced' societies, is, however, linked with an entirely material factor. This is the wealth of such societies, which has steadily grown from the earliest days of human civilization, as settled farming gradually superseded the nomadic hunting of game. As food supplies became more plentiful and more certain, one after another the nuts and roots, small wild game, wild leaves of diverse kinds – and insects as well – were, first of all, less highly prized, and then, not being customarily eaten, became taboo.

This is perhaps an example of the fixity of a custom *not* to eat a palatable and nutritious article of diet. L. Thon,[9] reporting from what was at that time the Belgian Congo, describes the well-organized system by which the local inhabitants caught termites, some of which they cooked and ate fresh, some of which they prepared for the market. This they did by drying them in the sun and then lightly frying them. In the month of May fried termites formed a lively article of trade in the town markets. A special variety of these insects, the denge-termites, may either be eaten direct or used as a source of a colourless oil of good quality, excellent for frying. Thon, in the course of his studies, purchased samples of the brownish, fried, aromatic-smelling termites offered for sale in the market and analysed them. He concluded that the analysis of 561 calories per 100 g., 36 per cent of protein and 44 per cent of fat was superior to most other animal foods.

In Japan, all sorts of insects form part of the diet, and are highly prized. Dytiscid beetles, which are common – but taboo – in the West, are caught in nets in Japan, the hard shell is removed and the beetles, after having been fried, are mixed with sugar and made into a sauce. Again, the maggots which are the larvae of *Vespa japonica*, Sauss, were at one time canned for distribution in the shops. They are also fried in oil and soaked in soya sauce or, alternatively, boiled in sauce. Grasshoppers are also roasted with soya sauce. C. L. Remington[10] visited the Nagano province of Japan where maggots

[9] Thon, L., *Bull. Agric. du Congo Belge*, 37, 865, 1946.
[10] Remington, C. L., *Entern. New.*, 57, 119, 1946.

and pupae of the wasp, *Vespula sp.*, are a favourite food which again are often preserved in cans and sold in the grocers' shops. Remington went into some detail in his paper in describing the various ways in which people who collect the wasp maggots do so without being stung. Of course, the consumption of silk-worm larvae is a well-entrenched custom in Japan. For many established matrons, mothers of families and respected members of their community, the savoury smell of the cooking larvae will bring back happy memories of their days as young girls in the silk factory. And besides, Bodenheimer in his monograph publishes the nutritional value of the larvae as food, including their content of vitamin A.

Entomophagy, the eating of insects, is merely one example of a dietary custom which is deeply entrenched among certain groups of the human population and rejected by others. Among Australian bushmen who live in arid, barren land where food supplies are scarce, a wide variety of insects are used for food. Sugar ants are particularly popular. The 'honeypots' – swollen abdomens filled with a nectar – are bitten off and the sweet taste accompanied by the sharp astringent after-taste of formic acid is considered particularly attractive. Witchetty grubs are famous as an article of diet eaten by aborigines. They have not been exactly identified, but are thought to be the larvae of a big longicorn beetle. The grub reaches a length of four or five inches and the thickness of one's finger. They are dug out of the roots of eucalyptus trees and eaten slightly roasted. Europeans who have tasted them speak well of their flavour. This insect, among a number of others, is so intimately a part of the life of the people that for some of them it has deep religious significance. These are members of the 'witchetty-grub totem', who consider witchetty grubs as sacred as their own ancestors.

Yet it is not only primitive peoples whose dietary customs include the eating of insects. In China, the Cantonese use several kinds of beetles as confectionery. *Hydrophilidae* are usually cheaper than *Dytiscidae*, and both are less expensive than giant waterbugs. And in earlier times the great King Asurbanipal in his capital near Nineveh served locusts on sticks just as we serve prawns or chipolata sausages; while Father Camboué[11] in 1886 reported that Queen Ranavalona II of Tananariva employed a band of women whose duties were to

[11] Camboué, R. P., *Bull. Soc. Nat. d'Acclimat de France*, 33, 168, 1886.

scour the fields for locusts so that the royal table might always be well supplied.

A community that belongs to a particular totem will not ordinarily eat their totem animal – this would be for them a monstrous act almost equivalent to eating their ancestors. Bodenheimer points out that the Australians of the witchetty-grub totem do in fact eat sparingly of witchetty grubs on the grounds that only by doing so can they gain sufficient strength to keep up the religious rites their totem demands. Industrialized citizens of the West do not belong to totems. They do, however, eat or abstain from eating particular foods for no clearly apparent reason almost as if the local customs possessed quasi-religious significance. For example, during a survey carried out in 1945, it was found[12] that English coalminers in the counties of Durham and Lancashire ate, on average, only 0·2 oz. of cheese a day. On the other hand, coalminers in Leicestershire and in South Wales ate 1·8 – 1·9 oz. a day, that is nine times as much or more. The Durham miners, when asked to explain their aversion to cheese, claimed that it was 'binding'.

The compulsion of custom is very much a characteristic of the family, group or tribe. Its hold is loosened when the group is split up and the bonds of familiar inter-relationship broken. Durham miners who leave home to work in a South Wales pit soon come to eat cheese without complaint. Masai herdsmen, transported to dig gold in Kimberley, eat what is provided by the commissariat, and manage without blood drawn from the jugular veins of their cattle.

Tribal habits in drink show a number of facets of the manner in which dietary customs affect both the happiness and wellbeing of different communities and their health. Many missionaries bringing Western enlightenment, and administrators bringing Western welfare, into Africa, have taken the view that the consumption of alcoholic beverages by the local inhabitants is bad and should be stopped. Many educated visitors to Africa have thought thus, but not all. For example, a clergyman at the start of the present century is quoted in these terms:[13] 'It is a very great error in my opinion, to assume, as many, even "Old Colonists", are apt to do, that this Kaffir-beer is simply and solely an intoxicating drink. It is, in my

[12] Pyke, M., *Proc. Nutrition Soc.*, 3, 134, 1945.
[13] Bryant, A. T., *A description of native foodstuffs and their preparation*, Govt. Printer, Pretoria, 1939.

view, much more than a luxurious and supererogatory beverage. It is rather a very admirable, very beneficial, even perhaps, very necessary form of food; and Governments in their legislation thereanent should recognize this fact, and aim rather at preventing its abuse than preventing its use.'

There are two good reasons to support this view. The first is social and the second nutritional. Various materials – sorghum, maize, millets, cassava flour with the addition of cereals, and plantains are used in the preparation of Kaffir-beers. Platt[14] quotes an eighteenth-century visitor to Africa as saying that in this country there are 'a hundred and a hundred' sorts of beer. The beverage is made often by partly germinating the cereal, mashing it in hot water and then allowing the whole lot to ferment. But the custom of beer-drinking in Africa as in countries of the West is very much more than merely an excuse to get drunk. Here is what Huntingford[15] wrote:

> The European who sees a Nandi continually getting drunk although he is at the same time short of food, does not realize that beer is a social necessity and not merely an enjoyment. If a Nandi cannot from time to time give a beer-party, even a small party, he will lose social standing; he will be considered mean and will not be asked by his neighbours to partake of beer. He will be, unofficially but none the less effectively, pushed out of his rightful place in the *koret* (i.e. parish).

And another observer[16] commented thus:

> [Beer drinking is] the people's only kind of entertainment, the chief break in the monotony of their village life, and, as in most other Bantu societies, the common, and sometimes essential way of fulfilling social obligations . . . it [beer] is carried to chiefs as tribute, used to reward labour, or given as an offering to spirits . . . Abundance of beer is the glory of a commoner's hospitality, or a chief's court. Without it tribal councils cannot be held, and marriage or initiation ceremonies do not take place.

But this dietary custom which compels the Bantu people to drink beer possesses a great deal more than social value, it has an important economic significance as well. Collective work is a striking feature of many of the less sophisticated communities in Africa. The beer-party

[14] Platt, B. S., *Proc. Nutrition Soc.*, 14, 115, 1955.
[15] Huntingford, G. W. B., *Colonial Research Studies*, No. 4, HMSO., 1950.
[16] Richards, I., *Land, labour and diet in Northern Rhodesia*, Oxford U.P., 1939.

44

is the usual form in which this collective effort is made. The men gather together to undertake the preparation of a garden for planting or to weed a field of grain. These tasks must be done quickly when the weather is right. The group of workers is cemented by beer-drinking, and regulated by the social ritual which surrounds it. The fact that the men like the beer they drink adds to its value as a social bond, but it is the compulsion of custom and etiquette that exerts the real force. At the beer-parties the work is done quickly and cheerfully, and the beer itself fortifies the endurance of the workers. Platt has observed that the traditional role of beer is strongest in the hill villages, less, so in the foothill villages, and least in the lakeshore villages where the increasing influence of Europeans has introduced the alien and characteristically Western mercenary attitude to life, so that men of the community work 'abroad' for money in mines and plantations.

The second significance of the drinking of Kaffir-beer is its contribution to nutrition. The beverage is much thicker than industrially produced Western beer. It provides energy; the germinated grain from which it is made also contributes vitamin C to the diet; and the fermentation leading to a growth of yeast in the beer contributes as well several B-vitamins in which the diet of the people who drink it may be lacking.

Here then we have a nice example of how much more complicated the science of nutrition is than the less perceptive students of conventional nutritional science sometimes imagine it to be. The patient brought into a hospital with severe head injuries received in a road accident who lies unconscious for months, is something with which such students can deal with confidence. The composition of the mixture flowing through the tube into the human body in the bed can be calculated with precision. It needs to supply the appropriate energy value and the appropriate balance of nutrients. But when the same scientific principles are applied to the same body when the man to whom it belongs is living a human life in an African village, there is much more to know. It is not enough to calculate then that the diet he is accustomed to eat is deficient in mineral content, and would be perfected by the addition of x milligrams of calcium incorporated in flour. The man may not eat bread. Nor is it good science to prohibit the drinking of alcohol, a potentially toxic substance which can be shown to intoxicate, if by doing so the man loses his friends, and if the community of which he is a member is unable to sow and till their land. And besides, people do not drink 'alcohol', but *beer*.

What holds for Bantu people living a village life in Africa, holds for all mankind. Dietary patterns are an important factor in their behaviour and reflect directly on their wellbeing. Dietary patterns can be changed, and the most potent cause of change is the creeping tide of industrialization which is steadily engulfing humanity. But although food habits can be changed, the strength of their roots must be recognized. Let us consider in this context, as perhaps a special case, the three main benign social drugs, alcohol, nicotine and caffeine, the addiction to which forms so striking an ethnological characteristic of modern Western societies.

To the eyes of the nutritional scientist, the consumption of alcoholic beverages can be undesirable. In excess, such drinking may lead to penury, cirrhosis of the liver (a scourge in France, where labourers drink continuously substantial volumes of wine), obesity (common among Bavarian beer-drinkers), and an increased mortality in road accidents. And the barley and other crops from which the drink is made are not available for general consumption. Yet the experiment in the United States of abruptly making the sale of such beverages illegal had disastrous effects on the social behaviour of the community, of far greater significance than anything attributable to the physiological and nutritional disadvantages resulting from the spirit-drinking which had gone on before.

The use of tobacco as a source primarily of the drug nicotine, is a firmly-fixed social habit among many communities all over the world, and has a particularly powerful hold on technologically advanced nations. This is so in spite of the fact that these nations are fully aware of the practical uselessness and the potential harmfulness of the custom. Its existence underlines what these communities often tend to forget, that social behaviour may more often be decided by emotion, custom and the blind forces of ethnology, than by reason. Reason informs civilized people that their food is drawn from all over the world, that the amount of food available for the world's population is inadequate for their nutritional needs, and that the area of land suitable for food crops is limited. Yet vast areas of good, well-drained arable land are devoted to a nutritionally useless crop. The United States might claim – although not all the world's citizens

46

would agree – that it is rich enough to be able to afford to waste enough land to grow 1,400 million pounds of tobacco a year. But what of India, where some 1,100 million pounds are grown, or China growing almost 1,000 million pounds? Rich countries such as Belgium, Canada, France and Germany, and poor countries such as Algeria, Bulgaria, Puerto Rico and Yugoslavia, all devote good land to the culture of tobacco.[17]

And not only does the growth of tobacco occupy land which could otherwise be used to grow food, but the method by which the drug it contains is taken into the body – the extraordinary social custom of sucking it into the mouth in the form of smoke – is almost the most wasteful method of using it that human ingenuity could have devised. If only the eighteenth-century custom of enjoying the pharmacological effects of tobacco in the form of snuff had continued to our own day, enormous acreages of ground would have been left free for food crops. The amount of nicotine in one cigar is sufficient, if absorbed efficiently into the body as snuff, to kill a man. The fact that it does not do so is because by smoking it the smoker allows most of the nicotine to go to waste.

The power of tobacco over quite sophisticated societies is as great as that of alcoholic drink. Britain, beleaguered in war, desperately resisting starvation at the risk of ships, aircraft, and men's lives, chose to limit food imports rather than restrict supplies of tobacco. In countries occupied by foreign troops during World War II, the currency which never lost its value, more precious than coin, and certainly more prized than notes – in Italy, France, Austria, Germany – was cigarettes. The most powerful corrupting influence in a society of men under the peculiar stress of prison is that of tobacco in the hands of the 'tobacco barons' who emerge to dominate their fellows.

That the compulsion of custom – especially when it results in addiction – is as important to human welfare (which comprises within its ambit 'health' as now understood) as protein, vitamins or any other nutritional component, must be accepted as a general principle. And the illogical customs of the West are as potent as any to be found in the East, in Africa or Australia. To alcohol and nicotine one can as readily add caffeine, the main pharmacological agent in tea and coffee. Written reference to tea dates back to the fourth

[17] US Dept. Agric. *Tech. Bull.*, 587, 1937.

47

century AD, and in the *Ch'a Ching* of AD 780 there is an illustration of a teapot very like those still used today.[18]

A nutritionist, whose scientific training often seems to imply that people eat to live, could again be forgiven for mistakenly believing that for civilized nations of the twentieth century tea is a trivial matter. The nutritional value of tea itself is negligible. The milk for which it provides a vehicle would be better consumed by itself, and the sugar which many people take with it can be positively harmful: it may contribute to obesity, it has been implicated in raising the cholesterol level of the blood,[19] and – being entirely lacking in protein, minerals and vitamins – it 'unbalances' the diet. Yet a moment's thought again shows that tea-drinking – and coffee-drinking as well, in communities addicted to it – may become a dietary habit so compulsive that to break it without understanding its strength can disrupt a whole society. Industries can be brought to a standstill if a 'tea break' is carelessly displaced and the workmen's nutrition, as well as many other facets of their life, radically disturbed. Politicians, who may be ignorant of science and nutrition but whose business it is to have at least a rule-of-thumb knowledge of the way communities behave, are well aware of the strength of the tea habit. Thus it could be argued that the compulsion of custom – the tribal devotion to tea – was to a degree responsible in 1773 for changing the history of Western man when in Boston the American colonists broke with the British crown on a fiscal principle arising from the import of tea.

The force of the same habit was apparent almost two hundred years later during the war of 1939–45. No sooner did a mechanized column of British troops halt in the North African desert, than, from each vehicle in the convoy, a man would come running with an empty metal drum. Into this went some sand and half a can of gasoline. A lighted match set the whole thing ablaze, the 'brew can' was set on top, and in a few moments every soldier was drinking tea.

Mankind is distributed widely over the surface of the globe. From Arctic lands in the north, through the temperate zone, to the equator, communities are to be found whose dietary habits are inevitably affected by the indigenous foods available in the areas they inhabit.

[18] Ukers, 'All about tea,' Tea and Coffee Trade J. Co., New York, 1935.
[19] Yudkin, J., *Lancet,* II, 155, 1957.

Nowhere, however, can it be assumed that men simply eat what they can get. No community is so poor or primitive but that – since it is made up of man who, wherever he may be found, is a subtle and complex being – the rules governing how the people eat exert a compulsive influence over *what* they eat.

During the three hundred-odd years during which scientific thinking has been used in the way we use it today, remarkable advances have been made. But these advances have always been on a narrow front. The exact sciences, physics and chemistry, based to a large degree on the precise intellectual tool of mathematics, have been most successful when used to attack a limited, well-defined target. The scientific study of biology too, has yielded fruitful knowledge when it has been restricted to clear-cut, manageable experiments. Darwin made precise records of the shape of the beaks of finches in the Galapagos Islands, Mendel observed whether peas were wrinkled or smooth. And in the field of nutrition, the productive studies were those in which diets of chemically-defined composition were administered to experimental animals – or men under controlled circumstances – and measured amounts of specific compounds (vitamin C or calcium carbonate) were added or withheld.

But now the science of nutrition is struggling to move forward into a new dimension: the dimension of human behaviour. This takes it beyond the limits of science and into areas of knowledge which have so far defied the exact scientist. The dictionary[20] defines 'politics' as 'political affairs or life'; 'political' as 'of public affairs'; and 'public' as 'concerning people as a whole'. In its real sense, therefore, 'politics' is whatever concerns the life of people as a whole. This, we know, although it has been studied by men of the first ability as a topic of high importance, has never been reduced to sufficiently manageable proportions to yield the decisive results of science. Anthropology, in the words of the dictionary, is the 'whole science of man'. Unfortunately, those who attempt to study even so limited an aspect of man as what he eats, are quickly compelled to admit that it has not yet been – and perhaps may never be – possible to comprise man within the ambit of science. 'Know then thyself,' wrote Alexander Pope,[21] 'presume not God to scan, The proper study of mankind is man.'

[20] *The Concise Oxford Dictionary, 4th ed.,* 1950.
[21] Pope, A., *An essay on man.*

In 1960 a scientific conference was held in Cuernavoca, Mexico, to discuss food habits and malnutrition.[22] Those taking part in this conference did so on the basis that the techniques of the social sciences and the information available from social studies and so-called cultural anthropology, had not been given an adequate place in planning national and international schemes to improve the nutrition of malnourished people. It was recognized that food habits were often deeply embedded in cultural tradition; and that superstition, religious belief and local custom all played a part in the resistance to change which the victims of malnutrition often showed to those attempting to introduce new habits and new foods to improve their lot. The proceedings of this conference showed very clearly the different degrees of precision and certainty between the biochemical knowledge of nutritional science, and the collection of observations comprising the corpus of anthropology and social psychology.

It was considered by some of the contributors to the discussion that food habits are especially firmly fixed, and that people who are transported to a new environment may change their language, their dress and their religion before they are prepared to change their diet. On the other hand, Margaret Mead quoted evidence to show that resistance to change might be strong or it might be weak. She suggested that when people had formed their habits in a loving environment, their behaviour was more firmly fixed in after-life than when they had been brought up under a system of rigid discipline. Italian immigrants to the United States retain Italian dietary customs. more tenaciously, it appears, than German immigrants retain theirs. Other contributors to the meeting put forward other ideas, for example, that Pavlovian conditioning played a part; that a man might feel that what he ate and the way he ate it was an attribute of his personality, to change which would be to change his idea of himself; or that there was a moral virtue in frugality, and that to pursue 'low living and high thinking' was a virtue even if it involved some measure of malnutrition.

Unfortunately the evidence for most of the deductions about how food habits are formed and how they become changed is unconvincing. Social anthropologists have collected much interesting informa-

[22] Burgess, A., and Dean, R. F. A., *Malnutrition and Food Habits*, Tavistock, London, 1962.

tion. Their subject, however, still bears as close a relation to history as it does to science. A politician can hope to influence social affairs to suit his will more effectively if he possesses a knowledge of the past history of his own and other nations; but, even if he calls his understanding 'political science', he cannot claim for such 'science' the precision of chemistry or physics. The nutritional scientist who aims to break the compulsion of custom must own an equal humility. There is, however, a group of observations which suggest with increasing certainty, that in one respect it is safe to predict the effect on existing custom of a particular influence.

The culture of Western nations in the twentieth century is based on science. The nations of the West and those who have accepted their intellectual ambience – the Japanese, the Israelis, the Soviet Union – have accepted the premise that this is an explicable, mechanistic universe. Rainbows, shooting-stars and earthquakes can be understood; other natural events, such as disease and famine, can be to some extent controlled. From this doctrine, which gradually took shape during the last three centuries, it was a short step, and one taken only during the past hundred years, to marry science with technology. The understanding of nature by the power of intellect was combined with the will – and with the ability – to do something about it. This culture is proving dominant over all others; its attractiveness and popularity are showing themselves to be irresistible to mankind.

The effect of science and technology on dietary customs in the West is instantly apparent. Remote tropical areas in the jungles of South America were once known as 'banana republics' because they served the highly capitalized food firms of the West as sources of supply of bananas, to be labelled and distributed to supermarkets all over the world. Baked beans, tomato ketchup, frozen chickens, frozen peas, white flour, granulated sugar, canned salmon, canned pineapple, fish fingers, Coca-Cola and Scotch whisky – all these are commodities of the twentieth-century West to be found being eaten and drunk by the nations of four continents. The culture based on science and technology has spread over the West, and is proving a potent force to change food habits even where other older cultures still persist, as they do in parts of Nepal, for example.[23] Gradually, nations and tribes, no matter how remote they may have been from

[23] Dart, F. E., & Pradhan, P. L., *Science*, 155, 649, 1967.

the main stream of Western thought, become addicted to Western food.

For the Western anthropologists who wish to study primitive ways, it becomes more and more difficult to find Australian aborigines eating their native diet. Eskimos no longer eat their traditional food, but, when they are able, turn to Western groceries.[24] The Bantu people who leave their villages to work in the mines and plantations become accustomed to Western food. The social forces which impel Europeans and Americans to embrace the products of large-scale food technology, that render the world-wide catering of the Hilton hotels irresistible from Istanbul to Amsterdam, exert the same effect over the emerging nations of Africa, Asia and South America.

Since history began, man has been subject to malnutrition and famine. Now that science and technology have made the world so small, famines in distant places, in Central America or India, can be seen by those who live in more fortunate lands, and today touch the conscience of wealthy, science-based nations. Nutritionists, using the special area of scientific knowledge upon which their expertise depends, reason that milk and meat, nutritious though they are, are extravagant to produce. In Guatemala, Scrimshaw and his colleagues[25] compounded a mixture of maize, sorghum and cottonseed oil, fortified with vitamin A, to possess a composition equal to that of milk. By skilful marketing, and because it resembled the pap customarily eaten in Central America, they achieved some success in persuading those in need to eat it. Its use did not involve too marked a change in custom.

To meet a need they fear will come – that is, Malthus' prophecy[26] of world famine – other scientists[27] have proposed that advantage should be taken of the efficiency with which leaves synthesize protein to supplement the world's food supply. The leaf protein is manufactured in a processing plant that expresses the juice, from which the protein is precipitated by heat. The product is a bland, green, cheese-

[24] 'Medical Survey of Nutrition in Newfoundland', *Canadian Med. Ass. J.,* 52, 227, 1945
[25] Scrimshaw, N. S., and Bressani, R., 5th Int. Congress Nut., Panel II, 20, 1960.
[26] Malthus, T., *An essay on the principle of population as it affects the future improvement of society*, London, 1798.
[27] Pirie, N., Rothamsted Expt. Sta. Rept., 173, 1952.

like substance. But so far, those in nutritional need have been reluctant to eat leaf protein. Two factors are against it. Its cost in money, if not in land, remains stubbornly high. More intractable than this, perhaps, it does not readily fit into any existing dietary custom, nor does it possess that ill-defined yet potent force to change accepted custom which is possessed by technological foods accepted by Western nations – such foods as ice-cream, fish fingers and cornflakes. In short, it is not to people's taste.

CHAPTER V

RELIGION, SCIENCE AND NUTRITION

The straightforward application of modern nutritional science to cure the present and impending problems of the world's malnutrition, is to calculate deficiencies in terms of nutrients, and then look round for food sources by means of which these deficiencies can be made good. This approach has indeed had some useful results. It is more economical in terms of human nutrition to dry the skim-milk left over from the manufacture of butter, and export it to India, rather than feed it to pigs. It is a valuable achievement to isolate leaf protein from pea haulms which otherwise would be wasted in the manufacture of frozen peas. It is a remarkable *tour de force* of biological virtuosity to isolate a strain of yeast capable of growing on hydrocarbon fractions which otherwise would only constitute a valueless by-product of the petroleum industry, and use the yeast, dried, to feed livestock, or even – after suitable preparation and in appropriately small proportions – as human food. Fish flour too can be prepared as an almost tasteless powder of high nutritional value to enrich the exiguous supplies of protein in the diets of poor, often overcrowded 'emerging' nations.

The main shortcomings of such straightforward scientific attacks on nutritional problems fall, however, into two groups. Firstly, the manufacture of these nutritional supplements – dried milk, fish flour, yeast grown on petroleum by-products – is only possible in a technological environment, just as the very knowledge of nutritional science itself derives from such a background. And this same technological environment has, to a major degree, given rise to many of the very problems which have to be solved. It is true that science, applied to agricultural production, has led to the development of fertilizers, insecticides, fungicides, new and improved strains of food plants and food animals, together with vastly improved machines and agricultural methods; it has enormously increased the productivity of the land. At the same time science, linked with technology, has – by making the world richer, in economic terms, and through the developments of drugs and the mastery of micro-organisms – made it safer, and in so doing has encouraged a steep rise in the world's population. Even if Woytinski and Woytinski[1] are right – and many sincere and thoughtful people believe that their calculations are wrong – that since 1850 to the present day the increase in food output has been proportionally more rapid than the increase in the human population, there still remains much that is wrong that should be put right. But apart from the deficiencies in even the current massive technological efforts, a second kind of obstacle related to what we have been discussing in the last two chapters is the influence on nutrition of men's religious beliefs.

When the scientifically trained Western nutritionist regards the malnutrition of millions of Indians in a country containing a fifth of the total cattle population of the globe, his initial proposal for increasing the happiness and welfare of the Hindus is to give them contraceptives and tell them to forget their religion and eat their sacred cows. But is this good advice, and is the Western scientist justified in giving it? After all, he has a religion too.

The exact origin of the prohibition against eating cattle in India is obscure but derives from a basic religious belief in the sanctity of life – not just human life, but the life of other creatures as well. 'Not to injure living things is good,' wrote King Asóka in his rock edicts of about 250 BC.[2] Although this proscription did not at first apply specifically to cattle, by the seventh century AD what is now the present orthodox Hindu attitude already existed.[3] The Hindus not only refuse to eat beef, but vehemently oppose the slaughter of cattle. They are prepared to go to almost any lengths and to use any means to protect them – by political, or legal methods, by the use of moral force and social persuasion, or, as history has shown, by the final resort of fighting.

The influence of non-Western religious feeling and belief on men's behaviour and hence on the way they view the environment which provides their food, can be followed particularly clearly in William Goode's[4] study of a number of separate races more primitive than

[1] Woytinski, E. S., & Woytinski, W. S., 'World population and production trends and outlook,' 20th Century Fund, N.Y., 1953.
[2] Davids, T. W. R., *Buddhist India*, Putnams, N.Y., 1903.
[3] Watters, T., 'On Yuan Chang's travels in India 629–645 A.D.', *Roy. Asiatic Soc.*, 1904–5.
[4] Goode, W. J., '*Religion among the primitives*,' Free Press Publishers, Glencoe, Ill, 1951.

those to be found in India. It is sometimes difficult for Western scholars to study ways of seeing nature other than their own, because of the intellectually destructive power of the scientific philosophy. Western science, as it spreads over the globe, can be seen to destroy the religions of more 'primitive' tribes and even to destroy the tribes themselves. 'Perhaps', wrote Goode in his book, 'if we continue our present increase in destructive efficiency, Western science will destroy all religion' – that is, other than the religion inherent in itself.

Biochemical analysis does not explain man's social behaviour, and a nutritional scientist is mistaken if he believes it does. Only by studying social behaviour, of which religion is a part, can any valid conclusion be reached. Driving forces of society, including the 'religious drive', are as real as the drive of 'hunger', even if scientists have not so far learnt how to measure them in quantitative terms. Religion is a philosophy or code with which the fabric of a community is permeated and by which its values are influenced. We ourselves 'believe in' science as we also do in economics. And economics exerts an obvious bearing on nutrition. This is strikingly shown when farmers – in the United States, France and other 'advanced' nations – are paid *not* to produce food in order to keep prices *up*! Before a Western scientist condemns the Hindus' treatment of their cattle as irrational, he must consider his own basic values. Goode puts the matter thus: 'It is only in societies where a maximizing of money means at the same time the greatest increase in means that a failure to work for the highest reward can be classed as irrational. And even then, if the values one holds highest are not to be achieved with money, such a pattern of action could not be classed as irrational.'

Goode studied five different primitive communities: the Tikopia, a Polynesian group; the Dahomey; the Manus; the Zuni, town-dwellers in New Mexico; and the Murgin aborigines of Australia. Although it may be considered justifiable to describe each of these as primitive, all follow complex systems of social behaviour, and their societies are in many respects more closely integrated than our own. Although in Western terms the Dahomey are poor, they nevertheless grind part of their newly-harvested millet into flour, mix it with water and sprinkle it over their ancestral shrines. At the same time, by a system of divination they discover whether strong drink or animals should be sacrificed at the shrines. The primary economic activity of the Tikopia is the production of food; nevertheless, not only is food used as a token, as a means of repaying various kinds of social obligations and as tribute to a chief – functions quite apart from its nutritional value – but it is also an essential means of making religious offerings. The Tikopia also observe food prohibitions, most of which are intended to induce turmeric, which they grow and then extract as a ritual colouring-matter, to become hard. Sugar and foods eaten in a mushy state must not be consumed during the time the manufacture of turmeric is in progress. The Zuni Indians observe most elaborate rituals in which complicated formal dances are danced and, again, various foods are used for religious and social, rather than for nutritional, motives.

Goode summarizes the situation thus: 'In each society a considerable amount of time, energy and wealth was allocated to religious activities. There are ceremonial and ritual feasts, objects are used in the actual rituals; there is a ritual destruction of objects, property, food, etc., or they are used up in the same manner; and at various periods many people are spending a considerable portion of their time in actually observing the religious patterns.'

In his final assessment, after tracing in detail the influence of their different religions on their social, economic and political behaviour, Professor Goode reaches the conclusion that for all these peoples – a dwindling residue still largely untouched by the Western philosophy of technological materialism – 'religion is action, not merely a set of philosophic speculations about another world . . . Religious belief demands action at every turn, action in this world, towards this world'. And turning from these 'primitive' tribes to the Western situation he writes: 'We are a generation lost, lost in the only fashion which is really troubling, that is, by our own self-judgement lost.'

It is important to recall that the Bible, in which is described the religion to which the peoples of the West are heir, starts out by commanding man to have dominion 'over the fish of the sea and over the fowl of the air, and over every living thing that moveth upon the earth. And God said, Behold, I have given you every herb-bearing seed which is upon the face of all the earth, and every tree . . . to you it shall be for meat'.[5] This Divine authority has had a profound effect on the present world food situation. The subsequent Mosaic prohibition against the consumption of animals which do not chew the

[5] Genesis, I, 28–9.

57

cud and divide the hoof – listed as the camel, rock badger, swine and hare; against the curious list of nineteen birds;[6] against fish not possessing both fins and scales; against winged insects which go on all fours – although locusts, grasshoppers and crickets were approved;[7] and against the weasel, the mouse, the lizard, gecko, crocodile and chameleon, have had much less effect on the behaviour of the technological West.

It is easy for the Western-educated observer to deplore primitive religions and the religions of the East with their proscriptions and regulations which, to the eyes of the scientific nutritionist, seem merely to interfere with the orderly ingestion of a nutritionally adequate diet. It seems perverse to hold that all living creatures are brothers if, by abstaining from eating them, protein-deficiency occurs. It appears irrational for a man to cultivate an irregularly-shaped piece of ground merely to avoid disturbing the burial-ground of his ancestors. And the Western creed that nothing should stand in the way of efficient scientific farming, adequately capitalized food technology, and the world-wide distribution of the products of large-scale food industry, is a powerful belief. The missionaries of this belief have been enormously successful in proselytizing less 'developed' communities wherever they may live, until there are few parts of the world – whether it be among the Eskimos of the north, the Equatorial Congolese, or the aboriginal inhabitants of Tasmania or Tierra del Fuego – where white flour, sugar and Coca-Cola cannot be found. Yet, even when these items have been replaced by canned orange-juice, dried skimmed milk and vitamin concentrates, perceptive nutritionists are aware that all is not well with the diet and health of many communities, even among those in the West. Indeed, the world as a whole may be moving towards an 'ecologic crisis', by which is meant that the very success of those whose belief is in reason may itself be destroying the natural environment upon which technological plenty depends.

Professor Lynn White, Jr., recounts[8] an apt story which illustrates the complexity of the situation. Aldous Huxley it seems was deploring the ragged and overgrown scrub in what had before been a grassy glade. He blamed the farmers who, for their own ends, had introduced

[7] Leviticus, XI, 20–3, Deuteronomy, XIV, 19–20.
[6] Leviticus, XI, 13–19, Deuteronomy, XIV, 11–18.
[8] White, L., *Science*, 155, 1203, 1967.

the disease, myxomatosis, to exterminate the rabbits which previously kept the brush in check. He overlooked the fact that, just as the farmers of the twentieth century had brought in the myxomatosis germ, so in their turn had the farmers of the twelfth century introduced rabbits as a domestic animal to provide protein for the English diet in 1176.

Throughout most of history, the winning of food has been one of man's main activities. Even in so-called 'advanced' societies, agriculture has been the chief occupation. In early days, the land was tilled by means of a primitive plough, which scratched rather than turned the ground. This could be pulled by two oxen at most, and in the light, rocky soils of the Near East and the Mediterranean it tilled the ground quite well (and still does) particularly when cross-ploughing was carried out. It was less satisfactory, however, for the wetter climate and heavier soils of northern Europe. There it was that, in about the seventh century AD, a plough of a more modern design with a blade to make a vertical cut and a mouldboard to turn over the sod was introduced. This was a remarkably efficient tool but its friction was so much greater than that of a scratch plough that it needed eight oxen to pull it. This technological fact had two important results. Firstly, farms were no longer square, but tended to take the form of long strips. The second result was that since no one man possessed eight oxen, several farmers combined together in a co-operative effort. Lynn White summarizes the effect of the change thus: 'Distribution of land was based no longer on the needs of a family but, rather, on the capacity of a power machine to till the earth. Man's relation to the soil was profoundly changed. Formerly man had been part of nature; now he was the exploiter of nature.'

Since the Christian era began, 107 kinds of animals and close to 100 kinds of birds have been exterminated.[9] The extinction of plants and lower animals is not so easily recorded, but probably greatly exceeds that of birds and mammals. The modern attitude is quoted by Cowan in these words: 'In general, we have acted with remarkable arrogance to the whole of Nature of which we are a part. Any part we do not want, we seek to destroy, completely and utterly. . . . With the destruction of each such "pest" by the use of the handiest, cheapest, most quickly acting pesticide, goes the destruction of anything else about which we do not care at the moment, or the eventual

[9] Cowan, J. M., *Nature*, 208, 145, 1965.

destruction of other things about which we may care but by such remote side-effects that the actual connection can be disputed.'

This is yet another part of the 'ecological crisis' which has affected the world's total food potential as well as almost every other aspect of the terrestrial environment. The effect on a comparatively isolated land mass such as the Australian continent may be seen to be especially dramatic. Elspeth Huxley[10] recently described it in this way: 'What has happened to the Aborigines is the same as what has happened to so many other species of Australian fauna: the white man has made fundamental changes in the habitat. As with bandicoot and wombat, scrub-bird and marsupial mouse, once the habitat goes so does the species. As individuals, humans are the most adaptable creatures on earth. As individuals they can change their diet, change their climate, change their habits and survive. But communities cannot; the community disintegrates into individuals who adapt.'

We 'believe in' rational scientific thinking and, as nutritionists, scientists can provide adequate protein of appropriate chemical composition and can prevent the diseases of malnutrition such as rickets, scurvy, beri-beri or kwashiorkor, and even obesity, which shortens the lives of thousands of middle-aged Western businessmen. Yet, just as the beliefs of the East deplete the soil through the numbers of sacred cattle, and the month of fast-days during Ramadan causes nutritional hardship to vulnerable members of the Muslim community, so does the faith of the West in science involve ecological crises with which the so-called 'advanced' nations have found themselves unable to deal. Something can be done to cope with obvious local effects: crop failures, attack by plant diseases, the emergence of a 'dust bowl', a forest fire or devastation by riparian flooding of the Mississippi here or the Yellow River there. These are crises easily seen and understood, dramatic in their impact. But the environmental changes of greater and more permanent importance take place so gradually and insidiously that they escape notice until their effects are irreparable and permanent. These are the direct results of the attitude of the West to nature – that is to the modern occidental religion. Contamination of the environment by the waste products of factories, kitchens and lavatories; the gradual invasion of the growing areas for plants and animals by highways and airfields, and by the sprawling blight that flows from the cities farther and farther into the

[10] Huxley, E., *Their shining Eldorado*, Chatto and Windus, 1967.

60

countryside and the oceans – these represent cumulative contamination of the environment. The indestructible wastes of technology such as beer cans and discarded automobiles, cigarette cartons and plastic bags, detergent foam and the ever-widening stain of sewage which, from an aeroplane, can be seen discolouring the seas adjacent to populated coastlines, are visible signs. But as well as these, there are radioactive dust in the atmosphere, and DDT and the like in the seas, extending to the farthest corners of the globe.[11] These are invisible but equally significant signs of the ecological crisis which do not immediately attract notice.

People's attitude to their ecology depends on what they think of themselves in relation to the world around them. Human ecology is, in fact, directly influenced by the current beliefs about the nature and destiny of man – that is, by religion. To the scientific eye of a Western observer this is clearly apparent in, say, India or the Middle East. Though not, to us, so clearly apparent, it is equally true of the West.

The victory of Christianity over paganism was indeed a major factor in the development of modern history. Christianity, developing as it did from Judaism, replaced the pagan idea of a settled world. In this world gods and goddesses – though differing from man by reason of their immortality – shared with him problems and quarrels, loves and hates between each other, and met him in not entirely unequal confrontation. Most important of all, these gods were parts of nature with its animals and birds, eagles, lions and bulls, love, wine, the oceans, the mountains and the great trees of the forest. The religion of the West replaced this by an implicit faith in personal spiritual progress. Christianity is a highly anthropocentric religion. Man is made in the image of God and everything on earth is put there for his use. It is a remarkable thing that even modern scientists, and such post-Christian thinkers as atheists, humanists and communists' (whose religious beliefs dispense with God and who pride themselves on their rational view of the universe) are equally anthropocentric. In spite of Copernicus, all the cosmos revolves around the minor satellite on which we live. Regardless of Darwin, we do not really admit that we are an indissoluble part of the rest of biological creation. Other religions can accept the birds of the air and the beasts of the field as fellow creatures. Western man knows that they are merely brute beasts.

[11] Sladen W. J. Z., Menzeit, A., and Reidel, W. Z., *Nature*, 210, 670, 1966.

In pagan antiquity every tree, every spring and stream, hill and rock, had its own *genius loci* – its guardian spirit. These were centaurs, fauns and mermaids, part human, part animal or fish, to show that Creation was one harmonious unity. Before a man cut down a tree, mined a mountain or dammed a river, he took steps to placate the guardian spirit of the place. Christianity destroyed all this, and left its converts free to exploit nature with indifference to the feelings of natural objects. The Christian idea of creation was, that the kindly Deity had given man dominion over nature. The study of nature from which science developed was started, under the title of 'natural theology', to discover further the nature of God.

At first nature was studied as a symbolic system by which God's mind could be understood. The moral virtues of hard work and diligence were written in the ant's lesson to sluggards. The rainbow in the sky was a coloured promissory note testifying to God's contract with man not to send a second flood. Rising flames were a symbol of the soul's aspiration. But this poetic, if pragmatic, approach to theology was gradually displaced by more sophisticated studies from which was obtained an understanding of natural phenomena little different from what we hold today. Up to the time of Newton and beyond, scientists explained the motives which drove them to work as a desire to unravel the mind of the Deity. The final stage of the progress of the Christian idea was the combination of science – the unlocking of the mechanism of Nature – with technology – the urge to master nature.

The effect of this Judaic-Christian dogma on the environment from which the dominant Western peoples must derive the food upon which the world's increasing population depends, has been profound. Two quotations from Professor White summarize the situation. 'We are superior to nature, contemptuous of it, willing to use it for our slightest whim. The newly elected Governor of California, like myself a churchman but less troubled than I, spoke for the Christian tradition when he said (as is alleged) "when you've seen one redwood tree, you've seen them all".' And later on, comparing the ideas of Christendom and its modern heretics, the rationalists and communists, with those of the older paganism: 'To a Christian a tree can be no more than a physical fact. The whole concept of the sacred grove is alien to Christianity and to the ethos of the West. For nearly two millennia Christian missionaries have been chopping down sacred groves, which are idolatrous because they assume spirit in nature.'

It is incontrovertible that the religious beliefs of the West have been responsible for the growth of science and technology, which are basically Western ideas. It is these manifestations of human thinking which have resulted in the very real ecological crises with which we are faced today.

It would be nonsense to suggest that the impact of Western religion, with its belief in man's right to a mastery of nature, has been all bad. The Western God has given the beasts of the field and the growing things to man as his servants and, by the use of his intellect, man has made them work hard. The effect of plant genetics to develop improved cereal grains has enormously increased the amount of corn produced from the land. Vast areas of North America where once buffalo roamed over the empty plains, doing little good to man, now yield ever-increasing quantities of wheat. The buffaloes have been exterminated, but huge populations of men in countries half a world away from the American prairies are fed. It is fashionable to sneer at intensive methods of livestock production; they are called 'factory farming', as if this made them less respectable. But their efficiency as a means of producing food is very high.

Technological methods of producing food have increased the amounts produced in the world year by year at a rate that has kept up with and may indeed have overtaken the rate of increase of the world's population.[12] Yet two things are wrong. The first is the so-called ecological crisis. The attitude that all nature is subservient to man is, as I have already described, destroying the environment in which men live. There are no signs that this destruction of the landscape of the world will hamper the amount of food the land produces. On the contrary, the increasing effectiveness with which machines tear up hedges, level valleys, flatten hills, drain marshes and irrigate deserts promises to accelerate further the efficiency of food production. Agricultural technology aims to convert 'the countryside' into an industrial food-production unit in the open air. The ecological crisis arises from the fact that industrial food production, like the industrial production of other goods, is something which cannot become part of the humane activities of man.

In the modern meaning of the word, a man's *occupation* is not

[12] Mayer, J., *Nutrition Rev.* 22, 353, 1964.

necessarily what he proposes to do with himself, it is rather what he is compelled to do so that at some other time he may live the way he pleases. Few men obtain pleasure from a factory, and equally few from a factory farm. And outside these areas where the few selected species are protected and propagated for food – selected strains of wheat, rice and maize, selected strains of potatoes, cabbages and peas, selected inbred strains of *Bos primigenius,* the archetypal ox, of *Sus scrofa* and *Sus cristatus,* the ancestral pigs, of *Ovis musimon,* the wild sheep – other kinds of plants and animals follow each other into extinction. It may not be true to assert that the Hindu, with his low money income and his unsatisfactory nutritional status is happier – and hence to argue that he is in the same sense healthier – than his financially wealthier, more adequately nourished Western brother who grows cattle to eat, not to reverence. While this may not be true, and while the defeat of squalor, want, ignorant superstition and the groundless fears which derive from it, are things of which the enlightened West can be justifiably proud, all is not well in the technologically developed countries. This is the ecological crisis of which I have written.

The second aspect of the Western religion of which a modern nutritionist must be aware is this. We have already discussed how he must take into account the fact that the people in whose nutritional welfare he is interested are something more than biochemical systems requiring set amounts of nutrition; he must, as we have seen, be aware of their customs and habits, of their superstitions and irrational beliefs; and of their religion – the basis from which it has developed and the consequences arising from its dogma and ethic. My argument is that the exploitation of nature by science is one of the consequences of the Western system of belief about what kind of world this is. And what arises from this exploitation is the large-scale industrialized system of food-production in which, by the use of science and technology, the world's supply of sugar and butter, wheat and green peas, bananas and poultry are gradually concentrated into very large commercial organizations.

These large establishments require great concentrations of capital which, in turn, depend on the accepted rules of economics. Early in the Christian era, usury – the lending of money only in return for interest – was believed to be wrong. This idea was derived from Judaism: 'Thou shalt not lend upon usury to thy brother; usury of

money, usury of victuals, usury of any thing that is lent upon usury.'[13]
Then came the long historical period which is only now ending, when
only by means of usury could wealth be gathered together in sufficiently large amounts to make it 'profitable' to grow and process
foods efficiently for distribution all over the world. If we accept, as I
assert we must, that the beliefs which underlie the behaviour of a
community constitute its religion, it is clear that in many technologically advanced countries a major part of their operative religion is the
conviction that it is 'only right' that an investor should obtain a
profit from his investment. Members of such a community actually
assume that since both food, and the supply of medical care and
nutritional council, are commodities, the people who wish to obtain
such commodities must pay the appropriate price for them. This may
seem to be obvious. Nutritionists have always taken into consideration both the nutritional composition of an article of diet and its
price, by which means they have been able to calculate the relative
cost of a gram of protein whether it is in the form of haricot beans,
mince or prime steak.

But although the need to take into account a community's beliefs
about money, as well as the laws of economics – which, while they
differ in many respects from the quite objective laws of the exact
sciences, possess at the same time a degree of validity regardless of
the outlook of the society upon which they are operating – may seem
to be obvious, it possesses complex facets which deserve to be
considered. The primitive peoples studied by Goode followed
religions different from our own. They used a significant proportion
of their food supply for religious purposes in spite of the fact that
they lived much nearer the bare subsistence level than we do. They
devoted a significant part of their working time to making turmeric
and to other entirely non-economic activities. They did this for
religious reasons. The nutritionist studying these people needs to
bear these facts in mind. But equally, although we in the West
prefer, when we can, to adhere to correct economic principles, and
although our religion has been the basis, first, of our scientific
achievements and, more recently, of our technological virtuosity, the
religious beliefs by which our behaviour is governed are changing.

Marxism, like Islam, is merely a Judaeo-Christian heresy. The
Marxists believe, as do the Christians, in perpetual progress, as well

[13] Deuteronomy, XXIII, 19.

65

as in man's right to exploit nature. Indeed, the Marxist abandonment of many of the conventional capitalist economic beliefs, including the 'lending of money upon usury to thy brother', is a reversion to a purer biblical ethic than the one which we ourselves profess. A nutritionist attempting, therefore, to remedy a deficiency of, say, vitamin A, has need to know, firstly, whether the religious convictions of the population in which he is interested allow them to kill sharks in order to obtain their livers. Next, he must discover whether or not the community believes that an enterprise designed to manufacture shark-liver concentrate can be blessed with prosperity only if it is operated at a financial profit. There may be three categories of community willing to run the factory without its making money. A primitive pagan tribe would be willing, if it knew how, to engage in a co-operative enterprise without thought of financial reward. A communist nation might do this too: to the communist religion, profit is sin. And a Western community converted to the principles of welfare will supply vitamins and much else without requiring profit.

Modern history has brought a change in the religious behaviour of the West. Consider the following passage:[14] 'The registers of the Parish of Greystoke, in the Cumberland Hills, during the year 1623 show that some forty people died either of starvation itself, or of what looks very like it. On 11th September, Leonard, son of Anthony Cowlman of Johnbie in that parish, was buried, "which child died for want of food". The next day Jaine, his mother, a widow, was buried also; she "died in Edward Dawson's barn at Greystoke for want of maintenance". Then on 27th September and 4th October, John Lancaster, another child, and his mother Agnes were buried too, deserted by the father; they also "died for want of food and means".'

This account is of a Christian community made up of men and women as kindly and virtuous as those who succeeded them three hundred and fifty years later. And England of the seventeenth century was not an impoverished land. There was no need for people to die of hunger. The reason they did was because of the beliefs of right and wrong and what was correct behaviour, upon which the social system of the times was based. This was, in fact, the religion of the nation. To say of a community that to its members property is sacred, is to use the word 'sacred' in its correct way. To take away a man's property is 'wicked', whether the taking is by a thief in the night or by

[14] Lazlett, P., *What the human race is up to*, p. 333, Gollancz, London, 1962.

the compulsory purchase-order of a Local Authority. It is a historical fact that in the seventeenth century these beliefs were firmly held. In the twentieth century such beliefs had markedly changed. Not only within a nation is Welfare – the sharing of food and goods of various sorts by the corporate will of the population operating through its system of government – an accepted principle, but between nations as well the sharing of food without payment goes on to a lesser or greater degree. The system is imperfect and capricious, but the fact that it is developing at all can be taken as showing a change in the ideas of morality held by technologically advanced peoples.

The dominant Western religion, teaching the supremacy of man and his absolute right to exploit his environment, has enabled food to be produced with matchless efficiency. Although there are – as there have always been – many people with too little to eat, there are now more than in any previous historical period with a plentiful and varied diet. Yet at the same time the breakneck spread of science-based technology and the parallel increase in human numbers have had bad results. Fire, and destructive agriculture, irrevocably destroy land; balanced ecosystems of plants, animals and soil are degraded to uselessness, forests are destroyed to make the Sunday newspapers, creatures become extinct for ever! At an increasing rate the ground is polluted and the air and sea as well, rivers become sewers which spread indestructible wastes to the remotest shores.

But at last, after having cut down the sacred groves for millennia, the people of Christendom are beginning to understand that they only live harmoniously on earth if they grant at least some measure of equality to the other living things around them. The new enlightenment is the acceptance of conservation as part of what modern nations recognize to be virtue. Like the conversion of Constantine to Christianity in the fourth century AD, the acceptance by President Theodore Roosevelt of the tenets of conservation, and his promulgation of the so-called 'Roosevelt Doctrine' in 1910, represented an important change in national morality. The people of the United States had, almost above all others, devastated the land in which they lived in the cause of economic exploitation. Forests, buffaloes, topsoil and Red Indians – all were cleared away for profit. The Roosevelt Doctrine recognized that forests, plains, animals and birds, mountains and rivers and the people living among them, were an inseparable whole; established public responsibility for the wise use of

67

the resources of great areas of countryside; and declared that science, the agency which had given technology its force, should be used as the working instrument to guide a public policy of conservation.

Theodore Roosevelt's policy was, like Constantine's conversion, the outcome of half a century of struggle in the political arena, as the old concepts of the private rights to all public resources were defeated in the devastated forest lands of America, and the utilization of water on the arid lands of the central continent passed into the hands of the nation. Fifty years later this evolution in the belief of Western nations about what is moral behaviour, though not by any means complete, is moving towards full acceptance. To technologically trained eyes, the world can palpably be seen as a closed ecological system; we are so obviously living in an overcrowded satellite circling the sun, that our newly won reverence for the sacred grove and the creatures of wood and stream is reinforced by rational self-interest. The scientific nutritionist, too, can see that to clear great plains so that huge and complex machines may have free run to garner wheat, or to level forests in Africa to clear a thousand-acre ranch for the culture of groundnuts as a source of cattle concentrate and margarine, can lead to disaster. This was the East Africa Groundnut Scheme of 1946. Religion, science and nutrition are indeed part of the same intricate interplay of which human behaviour is compounded.

CHAPTER VI

A LITTLE LEARNING

We have so far discussed the problems which may arise when anyone trained in the science of nutrition attempts to apply the facts of science to a human situation without taking proper account of what kind of a community he is changing. There is another area of uncertainty in which a nutritionist may become trapped. He himself may fail to comprehend the implications of the knowledge which has been codified as the so-called laws of nutrition; or, alternatively, he may have to persuade people who wrongly believe that they *do* understand, that, in fact, they are in error. Occasion may arise when it is very important to do this. Consider the history of Dr William Stark.[1]

Dr Stark was a true scientist, full of curiosity about the workings of nature and fully prepared to do something to find out more. Unfortunately much of the information which he accepted as the basis of his hypotheses was wrong, and so were some of the conclusions he drew. For example: 'Dr B. Franklin, of Philadelphia,' he wrote, 'informed me that he himself, when a journeyman printer, lived a fortnight on bread and water, at the rate of 10 lb. of bread per week, and that he found himself stout and hearty with this diet.' This is good so far as it goes, but even in the eighteenth century there was plenty of evidence available to show that *prolonged* subsistence on such a diet was inadvisable – quite apart from what common sense would say.

'He likewise told me', Dr Stark went on, 'that he knew a gentleman who, having been taken by the Barbary corsairs, was employed to work in the quarries, and that the only food allowed him was barley, a certain quantity of which was put into his pockets every morning; water he found at the place of labour; his practice was to eat a little now and then, whilst at work, and having remained many years in slavery, he had acquired so far the habit of eating frequently and little at a time, that when he returned home his only food was

[1] Smith, J. G., *The Works of William Stark*. London, 1788.

gingerbread nuts, which he carried in his pocket, and of which he ate from time to time.'

It is said that the Duke of Wellington, when accosted in the street by a gentleman with the words, 'Mr Jones, I believe?' replied, 'If you believe that you will believe anything.' Unfortunately, the capacity of apparently intelligent but only partially informed students of nutrition for unfounded belief appears to be almost limitless. Dr Stark believed things wildly more improbable than that life and health can be maintained on a diet composed only of gingerbread nuts.

'By Sir John Pringle,' he wrote, 'I was told that the inhabitants of Zephalonia, during some parts of the year, live wholly on currants. He also said that he knew a lady, now ninety years of age, who ate only the pure fat of meat.' And elsewhere he reported: 'Mr Hewson informed me that Mr Orred, a surgeon of Chester, knew a ship's crew who, being detained at sea after all their provisions were consumed, lived, one part of them on tobacco, the other on sugar; and that the latter generally died of the scurvy, whilst the former remained free from this disease, or soon recovered.'

The history of Dr Stark's nutritional studies is a good example of the peculiar dangers of half understanding. In his day, he was a pioneer of experimentation. Yet his own credulity allied with inadequate knowledge and – as the quotations from his book imply – a signal lack of good judgement, brought him to disaster.

It has been known since biblical times that different types of diet affect the health of the people eating them. For example, in the Book of Daniel there is the account of the young men whom Nebuchadnezzar took into his service. 'And the king appointed them a daily provision of the king's meat, and of the wine which he drank, so nourishing them three years, that at the end thereof they might stand before the king.'[2] When Daniel and his friends, Hananiah, Mishael and Azariah, were enlisted, he persuaded the officer in charge to allow them for a period of ten days to eat a more temperate diet mainly composed of pulses with water to drink. 'And at the end of ten days their countenances appeared fairer and fatter in flesh than all the children which did eat the portion of the king's meat.'[3] Dr Stark, like Nebuchadnezzar, proposed to study experimentally the effect of

[2] Daniel, I, 5.
[3] Daniel, I, 15.

different kinds of diet. With his head full of the remarkable stories which he had been told, his first trial was of the effect of eating nothing but bread and water. This he lived on from 24 June to 26 July 1769. Then he changed his diet but only to the extent of including sugar. On 11 of August he noted: 'I ate twenty-four ounces of bread and sixteen ounces of sugar, but the last part of it with great abhorrence. I now perceived small ulcers on the inside of my cheeks, particularly near a bad tooth, in the lower jaw, of the right side; the gums of the upper jaw, of the same side, were swelled and red and bled when pressed with the finger; the right nostril was also internally red or purple, and very painful.'

He had, in fact, given himself scurvy. The tragic feature of his situation was that, sixteen years before, James Lind, a Scottish doctor, had in 1753 described an admirable series of experiments from which he had correctly deduced the cause of scurvy, and demonstrated how it could be prevented and cured by eating oranges.[4] In spite of the obvious ill-effects of his injudicious procedure, Dr Stark persisted in his investigations, and put himself on to a diet composed of bread, water and olive oil. By 8 September he could hardly walk. But again he persisted in his faith that a diet of a few selected items was, as he had been told – or so he believed – capable of providing all the nourishment a man needed. Again he changed the mixture, this time to bread, water and milk. Soon this became bread, water and roast goose, followed by bread, water and boiled beef, and then bread, honey and rosemary tea. Poor Dr Stark! Honey to this day is believed to possess magical powers, and rosemary is sold in so-called 'health food' shops.

The last diet of all, after eight months' persistent experimentation, was bread, Cheshire cheese and rosemary tea. On 18 February 1770 he gave up the cheese, and on the 23rd of the month he died, a pathetic and extreme example of the tenacity with which people cling to ideas about diet which sometimes may be based on a little learning, but too often arise from irrational belief.

Let me quote one more example from earlier times before turning to modern instances. 'A gentlewoman', wrote Oliver Lawson Dick,[5] 'had a beloved Daughter, who had been a long time Ill, and received no benefit from her Physicians. She dream'd that a Friend of hers

[4] Lind, J., *A treatise on the scurvy*, 1753.
[5] Dick, O. L., *Brief Lives*,

deceased, told her, that if she gave her Daughter a Drench of Yewgh powdered, she would recover. She gave her the Drench and it killed her, whereupon she became almost distracted. Her Chamber Maid to Complement her, and to mitigate her Grief, said surely that could not kill her; she would adventure to take the same her self; she did so and died also.'

There are few topics upon which partial scientific knowledge has been deployed with more vigour and less judgement than that of the alleged nutritional superiority of brown bread over white. Before the invention of the modern steel roller mill, the production of really white flour was an expensive process. This white flour was more delicate in texture and flavour than the coarser brown flour used by ordinary people, and consequently it was popular with the well-to-do. It therefore acquired a prestige additional to its dietetic quality, and this prestige attached itself to 'whiteness'. Thus, when milling technology made it possible to produce very white flour cheaply, flour of extreme whiteness was manufactured. Remarkable technological and scientific efforts were devoted to the attainment of whiteness. Not only were all the darker parts of the wheat separated and removed, but the flour itself was bleached. Further efforts included the employment of plant geneticists in Canada and elsewhere who devoted time and trouble to breed a strain of wheat which should be free from the naturally occurring carotenoid pigments which are normally present, and which give a slightly creamy colour to flour.

We have already discussed some of the underlying reasons why people have strong emotions about food. Particularly violent sentiments are aroused in many parts of the world about bread, which possesses a central position in religious liturgy. Few people are able to discuss the composition of bread temperately, and this intemperance is often shared by those who use scientific information in their arguments.

The danger of a little scientific learning about bread is not that people are likely to poison themselves by reaching a wrong conclusion, or even to affect their health to any marginal degree. It is, rather, that confusion and error are always to be deprecated, and a student of nutrition who holds with violence to an untenable position about bread on allegedly scientific evidence is more likely to reach an equally unfounded conclusion on other matters of more importance. Not so many years ago I was acquainted with an Egyptologist from

72

the British Museum, a learned man distinguished in his own field, who was convinced – and I quote his own words that I well remember – 'white bread is poison'.

The reason why there is scope for false reasoning from scientific premises on the matter of white and brown bread is twofold. First is basic tribal emotion. The repetition of ritual slogans – 'bread is the staff of life,' 'to ask for bread and be given a stone (or cake or crumbs from the rich man's table)', 'to take the bread out of a man's mouth' – affects even the most conscientiously rational person. The second part of the reason is, that bread offers a good opportunity for applying science to answer an irrelevant question. There are several ways of viewing the question: 'Which bread is better, brown or white?' It might be construed to mean 'which contains more vitamin B_1?'; or, alternatively, 'which produces the most aesthetically attractive toast?'; or perhaps, 'which kind would better support the health of a poor man compelled to subsist on a diet solely composed of bread and jam?'

For five hundred years in England, delicate, soft, white bread was held in esteem and was eaten by those who could afford to buy it.[6] A coarse grey shirt keeps one as warm as, or warmer than, a delicate bleached white one. But a gentleman who has the money to buy the fine one will wear it. So it has been with bread. And with the coming of the nineteenth century, demand for white bread for the growing towns steadily increased. To improve the whiteness of their flour, bakers began to add alum, chalk or ammonium carbonate. In 1820, Wakley, the doughty editor of *The Lancet*, published a series of trenchant articles exposing these abuses, and defied the bakers to sue him for libel. These articles caused an immense sensation, and it is partly due to the fact that Victorian grandparents were shocked by what they read, that twentieth-century members of the intelligentsia continue to condemn twentieth-century white bread on insufficient evidence. Soon after Wakley's articles appeared, the use of the grosser flour adulterants was prohibited. But people had wanted a white loaf and they had wanted a cheap loaf. In the view of Professor McCance and Dr Widdowson, the nineteenth-century bakers probably satisfied most of their customers without doing them much harm; but in doing so they brought upon themselves considerable suspicion and

[6] McCance, R. A., and Widdowson, E. M., *Breads: white and brown*, Pitman, London, 1956.

abuse. The steel rollers and silk 'bolting' cloths of modern practice were introduced in 1870 to deal with the 'hard' wheat from America; and at the turn of the century the bleaching agents and chemical 'improvers' we discuss today came into use.

So we come to the present age of science. In this period, Sylvester Graham[7] was perhaps the first of the 'scientific' protagonists of brown bread. Next came Dr Allinson[8] who combined a vehement advocacy of brown loaves with teetotalism and anti-vaccinationism as well. By 1911, the discovery of vitamins provided ammunition for both sides in the debate on the respective merits of brown and white bread that continues to this day. For those people who are uncommitted in this extraordinary controversy it is astonishing to find scientists of considerable eminence taking up diametrically opposite opinions about the implications of what they conceive to be the facts.

There are two distinct lines of argument used by those who vehemently insist that brown bread is good and white bread is bad. The first argument, if it can be called such, is mere intuition. Alternatively, it could be called Dodoism. 'I must know best because I am older than you – and I say that brown bread is best' (or worst), depending on the particular Dodo. The second line of argument is analytical: brown bread contains more thiamine (vitamin B_1), riboflavin (once called vitamin B_2), niacin, iron, fat and protein, all of which in appropriate amounts are necessary for an adequate diet. In most instances, however, these scientific facts are irrelevant. A deficiency of thiamin is responsible for the disease beri-beri. In countries where beri-beri is endemic, the concentration of thiamin in the staple cereal may be crucial. For example, in the Philippines where beri-beri was a serious public health problem, the nutritional status of the population was significantly improved and the incidence of beri-beri reduced by the enrichment of rice with synthetic thiamin.[9] But in Britain and other Western countries, bread does not form a major proportion of the average diet; other constituents of the diet contribute thiamin, and beri-beri is never seen. In brief, assertions about the nutritional superiority or inferiority of individual constituents of a

[7] Graham, S., *A treatise on bread and breadmaking*, Light & Stearns, Boston, 1837.

[8] Allinson, T. R., *The advantages of whole meal bread*, London (undated).

[9] Salcedo, J., Bamba, M. D., Carasco, E. O., Jose, F. R., & Valenzuela, R. C., *J. Phillip. Med. Ass.*, 25, 519, 1948.

mixed diet can be applied usefully only when the composition of the diet as a whole is taken into account.

Of course, the same invalid arguments based on analytical figures used in support of brown bread can be used against it. For example, it contains more indigestible fibre and more phytic acid, a substance which may prevent the absorption of calcium from the gut: consequently – or so the pseudo-scientific argument goes – it must be a worse article of diet than white bread.

The weight of argument and incident about white and brown bread has been enormous. In the United States, the pharmaceutical industry manufactures vitamins for addition to white flour – but not oddly enough to sugar, where the nutritional argument is very much stronger. In Canada, an ingenious scheme was proposed to modify the technique of milling so that a particular structure of the wheat grain, the *scutellum*, which is especially rich in thiamin, passed into the flour stream rather than into the offal. In Great Britain, chalk is added to flour as well as vitamins to increase the calcium content of the diet. Protagonists on both sides – those in favour of white bread and those in favour of brown – have shifted their ground. Sometimes white bread is supported because it is claimed to be digestible, which is an important virtue; sometimes it is supported because it is what people want and freedom is a greater virtue even than good digestion. Brown bread has advocates claiming the scientific virtues of roughage, and others are prepared to fight for its wider distribution on the grounds of flavour. There have been accusations on both sides of bad faith, claims and counterclaims of widespread malnutrition. If evidences of visible malnutrition attributable, no matter how tenuously, to the consumption of the wrong sort of bread have been cited, they were called 'clinical signs'. If there was nothing to see in spite of the consumption of less nutrients than the amounts recommended by some expert body, the deficiency has been explained as 'sub-clinical'. Malnutrition from eating the less favoured type of bread was sought in man, in weenling rats, in puppies, in black-beetles.

Professor Garry of Glasgow University once wrote:[10] 'The whole problem of proper nutrition is so frequently bedevilled by ignorance, prejudice and fanaticism that it behoves every writer on the subject of food to exercise restraint, caution and rigid scientific integrity. He

[10] Garry, R. C., *Nutr. Abs. and Rev.*, 12, 332, 1942.

must be not an advocate but a judge, weighing all the evidence, guiding, and in a large measure protecting the jury, which is the general public.' Professor McCance and Dr Widdowson, after having read all there was to read, and having reviewed 720 references dating from 300 BC to AD 1957, came to the conclusion that the argument in the monograph to which I have already referred[11] had reached stalemate. It appeared that in the main the protagonists were, in spite of their own faith in their individual rightness, possessed of too little learning. So McCance and Widdowson pursued the matter in the only way useful to a scientist. They designed and carried out an experiment to get more facts.[12]

At the end of World War II, in 1945, there were in the cities of Duisburg and Wuppertal in Germany 150 children between the ages of 5 and 15 years living in orphanages. These children had been getting the standard food rations and, at the beginning of the study, were about 9 per cent underweight when compared with American children of corresponding ages. The experiment was to replace the rather scanty German bread ration by an unlimited supply of one or other of five different breads. The kinds of bread selected were made from whole wheat flour; from flour of 85 per cent extraction – the type of flour used in Great Britain during the exigencies of World War II; from white flour of 70 per cent extraction; and, finally, from white flour to which the vitamins thiamine, niacin and riboflavin had been added, as well as iron to raise the amount of all these nutrients to the level at which they occur in whole wheat flour.

The children were carefully examined, weighed, measured and X-rayed before the trial began. Then the amounts of bread they ate, together with every other item of their diet, were recorded. The main articles in this diet derived from the German rations were vegetables, soups and potatoes, and about 3 oz. of milk. Because of the comparative shortage of food at the time, the children ate large amounts of the additional bread supplied to them. It was, therefore, reasonable to expect that any differences in the nutritional value of the breads would be reflected in their health and growth during the full year the trial continued. Nothing of the sort happened. The nutritional status

[11] McCance, R. A., and Widdowson, E. M., *Breads: white and brown*, Pitman, London, 1956.
[12] Widdowson, E. M., & McCance, R. A., Med. Res. Council, *Spec. Rept. Ser.*, London, 287, 1954.

of the children in all the groups improved equally. Their heights and weights gained at an equal rate, and this rate was faster than those of American children of comparable ages. This was because they were undernourished when the experiment began, and had therefore some leeway to make up. At the end of the year, there was not a penny to choose between the performance of any of the groups, regardless of whether their diets had contained white bread, brown bread, or white bread reinforced with vitamins and iron.

In assessing the results of their work, McCance and Widdowson wrote: 'If one of the groups had made less progress than another it would in a way have made this a more satisfactory experiment because, if it had shown conclusively the advantages of, let us say, wholemeal over white flour, the results of . . . studies on growing rats would have been shown to apply to children. Experiments, however, are not made to give satisfaction but to win knowledge. What knowledge had been won? . . . Not of course that there were no nutritional differences between the breads, but only that within the period of a year and under the conditions of this experiment no differences had been demonstrated between their nutritional value.'

In the 1930s, there were a number of people who, basing their argument on what they believed to be scientific truth, were responsible for increasing the number of British children contracting tuberculosis of the bone, and of adults contracting undulant fever, because of their involvement in a violent controversy about the pasteurization of milk. These people preached the purported scientific 'truth' that cow's milk had been specially created as a natural food for man, and that any interference with the state in which it leaves the udder is harmful, if not altogether sinful. Professor Kon[13] has summarized the situation thus: 'What is a natural food for an omnivorous animal such as man I have never been able to understand, nor could I perceive why it should be more unnatural to heat a cow's milk than to cook her flesh.'

Milk is an excellent food for man, and it is an equally good food for bacteria. Once inoculated with bacteria, which find it an admirable culture medium, it can become a dangerous vehicle of infection, particularly if a significant period of time elapses between the original inoculation and the eventual consumption of the milk. Organisms can

[13] Kon, S. K., *Nutr. Rev.*, 25, 129, 1967.

find their way into milk from the cow herself, from a dirty udder, from the dirty hands of milkers, dirty milking machines, pails, utensils, bottle-filling machines or bottles, from the air, from infected people coughing into it, or from flies settling on the pails or on other surfaces with which it may come in contact. Apart from salmonellae and staphylococci causing food poisoning, milk may be infected by organisms causing tuberculosis, diphtheria, scarlet fever, streptococcal sore-throat and undulant fever. Why then should any rational individual wish to expose his fellow men and particularly the children of the community, when the organisms causing this entire formidable battery of illnesses can be destroyed by the controlled heating of the milk to 72°C. (160°F.) for 15 seconds?

A little learning can indeed be a dangerous thing and, such as it was, it was deployed and entrenched in a stubborn rearguard fight which extended over many years. Immunity to a disease, the opponents of pasteurization asserted, is developed by having experienced the disease and survived it. True, Eskimos and Sherpas in the Himalayas who have little contact with civilization and are, therefore, deprived of the advantage of having had repeated colds and an attack of measles, catch cold immediately when they meet men from the cities of the world and die in epidemics of measles. Consequently – so runs the half-informed argument – children will grow up with greater resistance to the dangers of life if in their youth they have been exposed to milk supplies infected with homoeopathic doses of tubercle bacilli.

Professor G. S. Wilson in his monograph on the pasteurization of milk[14] listed nine separate lines of argument, all purporting to be based on scientific evidence, which had been put forward by opponents of the process, and dealt summarily with them all. The remarkable feature about this is not Wilson's diligence in pointing out the falseness of these claims, but rather the persistence and perversity which moved their proponents – who gained no profit from their energies, and who presumably meant no ill to their fellows – to take the stand they did. 'Pasteurization diminishes the nutritive value of milk,' was the first argument. 'It affects the taste and palatability, it affects the cream line, it affects the acidity, it reduces the amounts of calcium and phosphates, it causes protein to coagulate at five degrees higher temperature, it destroys vitamin C, B-vitamins, vitamin D and

[14] Wilson, G. S., *The pasteurisation of milk*, Arnold, London, 1942.

vitamin E.'[15] To this broadside, Professor Wilson replies that the first three points are irrelevant, the fourth – about calcium and phosphate – untrue, the fifth irrelevant, and the last largely untrue, and, where true (some vitamin C *is* lost) unimportant, since adults do not depend on milk for their vitamin C, and children are the better for safe milk and orange-juice.

Next, the objectors complained that 'pasteurized milk may diminish resistance to disease.' There is no evidence for this as a general assertion, and the idea of giving children tuberculosis by feeding them infected milk, so that those who survive may be the tough ones, is grotesque. 'Pasteurized milk interferes with the proper development of the teeth and predisposes to dental decay,' was an assertion based on half understanding an investigation of a medical research worker[16] who reported on the excellent teeth of boys in an institution where the milk was not pasteurized. But there was no equivalent group of boys drinking pasteurized milk to compare with the others.

'Pasteurization leads to the distribution of dirty milk and diminishes the incentive to produce clean milk,' was a frequent argument. This too is without merit, unsupported by evidence; and is contraverted by the fact that dirty milk may be tainted, and may contain organisms resistant to pasteurization which, while incapable of causing disease, will make the milk go bad. No sensible dairyman with an interest in the success of his business would want to pasteurize dirty milk.

And besides the main barrage of misguided argument there was as well – and in recent times when scientific information was plentiful – a scattered fusillade of even less well-conceived objections. These ranged from allegations that pasteurized milk would diminish human fertility, and thus lead to a fall in the birth rate; that it destroys hormones and enzymes, and thus takes 'life' out of milk – whatever that means; all the way to the assertion that milk pasteurization must be bad because it is not recommended by the Pasteur Institute! It should perhaps be said about this last remarkable argument that, firstly, the main business of the Pasteur Institute is the treatment of rabies, for which it was established, and secondly, that it is not true.[17]

[15] Heap, J. H., *Home Farmer*, 6, No. 3, 20, 1939.
[16] Sprawson, E., *Proc. R. Soc. Med.*, 25, 11, 1932; *Scot. J. Agric.*, 16, 23, 1933; *Brit. Dent. J.*, 56, 125, 1934.
[17] Kon, S. K., *Nutr. Rev.*, 25, 129, 1967.

It seems impossible to justify the opposition to pasteurization on rational grounds. Perhaps the most irrational reason is the easiest to understand. A man who claims that heating milk destroys the 'life' in it is responding to a deep-rooted mystical feeling – an emotion. But a man who talks of the coagulation of protein and the loss of phosphates is apparently citing science, and, by implication, using reason to justify his argument. To deal with such objections (in deference to which the use of pasteurization to make milk safe from the germs of disease presenting real and immediate danger was deferred in Great Britain and elsewhere for more than a decade) elaborate trials were carried out. In the United States, Frank and his colleagues[18] surveyed 3,700 children given pasteurized and unpasteurized milk. Leighton and McKinley[19] in Scotland studied two groups, each comprising 5,000 children. An experiment in England[20] covered a total of 8,000 children. All these laborious investigations failed to show any difference in the nutritional value of pasteurized and unpasteurized milk as measured by their effect on the growth and health of children. Yet in spite of the massive deployment of diligent effort, in spite of the absence of evidence of harm, the emotions of the objectors – all citizens of a scientific age living in a technological community – were only imperceptibly modified. Even among scientists it is said that one must not expect one's opponent to be convinced by scientific evidence against his will, one can only wait for him to die.

The argument about the value of milk pasteurization is now ended. In Great Britain, the logic of the process was finally accepted by the nation in World War II – as the logic of votes for women had been in World War I. The conclusion came when the British citizens found that American soldiers based in England were not permitted to drink the local milk-supply because no assurance could be given that it was properly free from infection.

The danger of reviewing the ill-effects of the misuse of incomplete knowledge and defective understanding in the past is, that it may lead to a smug assumption that we are too wise to fall into the same kind of errors in our own enlightened times. The value of looking

[18] Frank, L. C., et al., *Pub. Health Ref.*, Wash., 47, 1951, 1932.
[19] Leighton, G., and McKinley, P. L., 'Milk consumption in Scotland', Dept. Health, Scotland, HMSO, 1930
[20] *Milk and Nutrition*, Part II, Paynder, 1938; Part III, 1939.

back is to clear our vision to see our own equal danger of blindness. One striking historical fact is the long duration of mistaken ideas based on half-science. The fervent faith in the virtues of animal manure and the 'humus' it is believed to contribute to the soil, derives from a mistaken idea that plants derived their nourishment from humus. This so entered into the beliefs of people who considered themselves to be educated, that it persists even to this day; and in spite of the fact that Justin von Liebig demonstrated in 1840 that the substance of green plants was in fact made up mainly of the carbon dioxide gas they obtain from the atmosphere.[21] Similarly, there are people who still assert that canned foods are dangerous and lacking in nourishment. This idea dates back to the early days of canning when the process was merely technological and before the science of bacteriology had been discovered. Because the importance of applying sufficient heat to destroy micro-organisms in the centre of a can was not understood, the early history of canning records stories of too large cans being processed at too low a temperature for too short a time, rendering the food in them uneatable when the cans were opened. All this happened in 1845! And yet, the test for adequate sterility of corned beef, based on the 'scientifically' acceptable test that an infected can would bulge if it was incubated, was found in 1965 in Aberdeen not to be scientifically valid after all – and a typhoid epidemic broke out.

The big problem of the modern age is to try to ensure that the principles of nutrition as a whole are understood by those whose business it is to deal with the questions of human hunger and human wellbeing. If, through having only half understood the facts, and by possessing little real knowledge of their implications, the wrong conclusions are drawn, then indeed a little learning can lead to dangerous decisions. Misconceptions about the fluoridization of drinking water or the influence of mutton-fat on the incidence of coronary heart disease may be serious; but to be mistaken by millions about how many people are starving in the world may distort the entire public policy of nations.

It is a commonplace to read that a half – or sometimes, depending on the author, three-quarters – of the entire population of the earth are underfed, or sometimes, so it is stated, starving. This assertion is

[21] Liebig, J. von., *Die Chemie in ihrer Anwendung auf Agricultur und Physiologie*, 1840.

professedly based on scientific fact. In 1966, Dr B. R. Sen, Director General of the Food and Agriculture Organization of the United Nations reported that[22] 'the world food situation is now more precarious than at any time since the period of acute shortage immediately after the Second World War.' He also stated that because of 'widespread drought', food production in 1965–6 was the same as in the previous year 'when there were about 70 million less people to feed'.

Drought in some parts of the world has a more serious effect on food supplies than in others. For the world as a whole, however, upon, which the 70 million new people arrived, the rainfall from year to year is much the same. The water evaporates from the sea and, in due course, falls down again. World food supplies, although they fluctuate have increased steadily and, indeed, remarkably fast throughout the last hundred years or more of science and technology. The dedicated officials of FAO may have let their concern for those suffering from want most acutely, cloud their vision of the total situation with which they were required to deal. Their own figures showed that whereas food production in Latin America fell by 2·5 per cent in 1966, and production in Africa fell by 2 per cent, in North America the production of food continued to increase more rapidly than the increase in population numbers, and was 5 per cent greater than in the previous year.

The human predicament throughout history has always been a difficult one, ever since the first members of *Homo sapiens* found themselves in competition with the wild beasts who peopled the earth before them. It is important, however, for Dr Sen and the enlightened members of the scientifically-oriented communities whose spokesman he is, to keep a cool head and to assess the evidence which science provides as a whole, before deciding whether the time has come to prophesy doom. In assessing the adequacy of the world's food supply and judging the consequent nutritional status of mankind, a certain depth of vision is necessary. For example, according to the statistics of FAO itself the food production in the world as a whole increased by 32 per cent in the ten years from 1956 to 1966, and the amount of food available for every member of the growing world population increased by 7 per cent. It is true that in some countries, notably those in Europe and in the Soviet Union, food production increased

[22] *State of food and agriculture 1966*, FAO, Rome, 13 Oct. 1966.

much faster than population, whereas in others – Latin America and Africa for example – the advance was less. But even there, agriculturalists more than held their own over the decade. Mankind has never found it easy to feed itself; the problem tends to become more difficult in the new dimension of the world, which is diminished in size by the technological revolution in rapid transport, and instantaneous communication, and in which each part is increasingly dependent on such ever-closer-knit links of international technology as oil and drugs, complex machines, and specialized food technology. It is dangerous for world-organizations to be mistakenly complacent, but it is equally dangerous for them – through partial knowledge and inadequate thougnt – to be emotionally alarmist. The problems to be faced are real and very difficult, but they require much learning, not little and partial, for their solution.

'To the unknown men and women in all parts of the world who must apply this fundamental knowledge of nutrition in the day-to-day task of treating and preventing malnutrition': so reads the dedication of a treatise on nutritional science published in 1966.[23] A description of how difficult it is to apply such scientific methods appears later in the same volume.[24] And it is of these difficulties that the people who make pronouncements, give sermons, appeal for funds, or influence international policy, must be fully aware. To start with, statistics of food supply need to be examined and understood. It is never easy to find out how much people have to eat. Even if some sort of an estimate is available of the amounts of different foods brought into a country, and of the quantities grown within its own territory – a particularly difficult estimate to make if people grow food merely for their own use – it is also necessary to find out how effective the system of transport is, whether much of the food is destroyed by vermin while in transit or being stored, and – perhaps most important of all – whether people have sufficient money to buy such food as is available. There are laws of economics which, while not possessing the absolute validity of scientific laws, nevertheless operate according to certain principles. And one of the principles of economics unfortunately is, that in times of scarcity prices rise, and when prices rise there are always people to be found manipulating affairs to make themselves a

<hr />

[23] Beaton, G. H. & McHenry, E. W. (eds.), *Nutrition. A Comprehensive Treatise*, Vol. III (Academic Press), New York, 1966.
[24] Ibid., Schaeffer, A. E., 'Assessment of nutritional Status,' p. 217.

profit. Nutritional scientists ignore money at their peril. A popular British myth holds that the intellectual brilliance of the scientific control of our national diet during World War II was solely responsible for the improvement in nutritional wellbeing that took place during the war, This is only half true. Of equal significance was the fact that during World War II the British civilians were busily at work earning good wages.

There are a number of ways of finding out what people get to eat. One way is to ask them. This, in technical terms, is called collecting a 'dietary history'. Investigators can cover a lot of ground using this method, but the accuracy of their results is low. An alternative process is to collect information of a weekly food-budget – that is, to prepare a list of every item bought or used by a family during seven days. This is much more difficult to do. It involves an investigator spending so much time at each house that he or she is almost living there. The very fact of this close attention may itself alter the diet. An even more precise method of measuring what people eat is to weigh out two portions for every person in the survey and take away each second portion to analyse it. In practice this can be done only under quite special circumstances and for a very few selected people.

As soon as one stops to consider how statistics of food-consumption are obtained, how inaccurate the figures must inevitably be, how difficult it is to find out how much food is wasted – or how much food the people being surveyed get, but say nothing about – the more discriminating one must be in comparing the estimates of the amount of food eaten and its calculated nutrient value, with estimates – no matter how determined by the experts – of the requirements of each nutrient for health.

Without vitamin C a man develops scurvy, without niacin he gets pellagra; a child without protein does not grow and may have kwashiorkor; without calories, people starve. Nutritional authorities have drawn up tables to show how much of each nutrient different kinds of individual need to protect them from these ills. The United States estimates[25] are for those amounts 'which will maintain good nutrition in essentially healthy persons under current conditions of living'. The British figures[26] 'are believed to be sufficient to establish and maintain a good nutritional state in representative individuals in

[25] US National Research Council, Food & Nutrition Board, 1963.
[26] *Nutrition Committee Report*, 1950.

the groups concerned'. The figures with which we are so frequently horrified, which are often used as a measure of the number of people in the world who are 'undernourished' or 'hungry' or – sometimes – 'starving', are all those whose consumption of nutrients falls in any respect short of one or other of the official tables.

A little learning is a dangerous thing. Those who have more – the men and women who are called on actually to apply scientific knowledge to a real situation – find themselves using supplementary tables. Such a one, called by Schaeffer a 'suggested guide to the interpretation of nutrient intake data', provides estimates below which recognizable deficiency symptoms can be expected in fact to appear. These estimates are not 10 per cent or 20 per cent or even 30 per cent lower than the official figures. For many nutrients they are only one-half or one-third as much. It is a good idea to eat what the US National Research Council or the British Medical Association say you should; but the people who list all those who fall below the recommended values, by no matter how little, as 'undernourished', 'hungry' or 'starving' are crying wolf where no wolf may be.

CHAPTER VII

SELF-DECEPTION AND SELF-INTEREST

Samuel Madden, who died in 1769, wrote: 'Words are men's daughters, but God's sons are things.' This idea was used later by Dr Johnson in the preface to his English Dictionary when he put the same thought thus: 'I am not yet so lost in lexicography as to forget that words are the daughters of earth, and that things are the sons of heaven. Language is only the instrument of science, and words are but the signs of ideas: I wish, however, that the instrument might be less apt to decay, and that signs might be permanent; like the things which they denote.'

Nutrition is a science, and science deals in precise observation and exact measurement. But when these measurements and observations and the conclusions drawn from them are set down, they are set down in words. And words are slippery customers, hard to hold down to a clear and single meaning. Besides this, they possess a flavour over and above their meaning. This flavour affects scientists just as it does other men. 'Plump' has good and agreeable overtones; 'obese' is bad and pejorative. But besides the inexactness and partial feelings attaching to the words in which nutritional conclusions are reached, the nutritionists themselves are also human and, as such, are liable to subjective bias. No scientist can deny that at some time in his career he has carried out an experiment, not to determine the truth, but to prove what he wanted to prove. Honesty is as hard to achieve in science as in any other honourable human activity.

The word 'vitamin' has a good sound. The discovery of vitamins in 1912[1] made a great stir in the scientific world. The idea that the *absence* of certain special and peculiar chemical compounds from the diet could cause ill-health and disease, came as an intellectual shock to a generation brought up on the belief – established by the work of Pasteur and his successors – that disease was caused by the *presence* of biological agents, also only in very small amounts. Almost at once people began to believe that, because a patient with beri-beri, pellagra, scurvy, xerophthalmia or rickets became better and healthier

[1] Funk, C., *J. State Medicine*, 20, 341, 1912.

by consuming one vitamin or another, this implied that ordinary people, not ill but afflicted by the minor disabilities of civilized life – headaches, indigestion or the vague and ill-defined but popular conditions of 'lassitude', 'debility', 'stiff joints' or 'sluggish liver' – could enjoy what even textbooks of nutrition described as 'positive health', if they added *more* vitamins to the diet they were already eating.

The idea of 'positive health', widely held as it once was by nutritionists, is a treacherous one. It is difficult to determine with any degree of precision what is the precise amount of any particular nutrient needed to prevent even the very slightest signs of malfunction or ill-health appearing. It is simpler to measure the amount of, say, the vitamin, thiamine, needed by rats. This can be done by taking a uniform group of young rats, feeding them a diet containing graded, measured amounts of thiamine, and watching what happens. This is much more difficult to do with people. But even when it *is* done, the interpretation of the results is by no means easy and leaves much to the judgement – and prejudice – of the investigator. And this is the difficulty. A nutritionist who is convinced that an ample supply of vitamins is a good thing, even though 'in the present state of knowledge' there is no objective evidence to support his opinion, cannot absolutely be gainsaid. It follows, therefore, that a food-manufacturer anxious to sell a product rich in thiamine, can claim that the people who eat it will feel better if they do so. He may, indeed, come to believe seriously that this actually happens, and find sincere and conscientious men to support him in his belief. But consider the real difficulties involved in fairly coming to the truth and making a balanced judgement.

If there is a radical lack of thiamine in a diet that provides enough, or almost enough, to eat, beri-beri occurs. Apart from the physical symptoms of this disease, which need not be described here, the frame of mind engendered by beri-beri has been described[2] as a feeling that 'it is better to sit than to stand, it is better to lie than to sit, it is better to die than to live.' And these feelings have been expressed by men subjected in the cause of science to experimental deficiency of thiamine. 'The deficient men were uniformly apathetic, disinclined to either physical or mental effort and depressed. All time free from tests and other set features in the programme was

[2] Keys, A., *et al.*, *Amer. J. Physiol.*, 144, 5, 1945.

devoted to lying silently in bed. . . . It is noticeable that their lack of desire to eat was not limited to the experimental diet; for example, they were only mildly intrigued by the thought of beefsteak or fresh vegetables, which they had not eaten for seven months.' It can, therefore, be said that among the symptoms of beri-beri, which is due to a shortage of thiamine, is an overwhelming feeling of gloom and despair. To what extent, then, can it be claimed that groups of people who are gloomy and despairing are suffering from a shortage of thiamine?

The first answer is that vague symptoms of this sort may indeed be an indication of malnutrition. Nutrition is, as it is the purpose of this book to show, only one of the factors to be considered when the human condition is in question. An impoverished, undernourished community may be debilitated by a combination of malaria, vitamin deficiency and intestinal parasites, and, as well, may be suffering from what Leighley[3] has called 'poverty of the spirit' from having lived for generations at a precarious level of bare subsistence. This condition is not restricted to poor countries in the remoter parts of Africa. As Leighley pointed out, in the southern United States honest if misguided observers, seeing populations attempting to live on inadequate incomes and a consequently unsatisfactory diet, have come to the conclusion that they were lazy, good-for-nothing people, whom it would be unavailing to help since the money would only be wasted. Under these circumstances, depression, gloom and an inability to settle down to work can indeed be symptoms of malnutrition and may be caused specifically by a shortage of thiamine. When this is so, however, it is almost certain that clinical signs of vitamin deficiency will also be found if the nutritionist goes out of his way to look for them. It is also likely that if thiamine is added to the diet – for example, by incorporating it in bread or enriching the rice – there will be a recognizable change in the health of the population.

On the other hand, it is very much less likely that the lassitude and lack of appetite felt by a bored, middle-class lady in a prosperous civilized community is due to thiamine deficiency. Yet it is easy to argue that it *may* be. And the argument seems more plausible when the individual supporting it has an interest in the matter. This interest may merely be that of a dietician trained to look for deficiencies in diets. Or it may be a financial interest in the sale of

[3] Leighley, H. P., *Science*, 156, 1312, 1967.

vitamin tablets, wheat germ or dried yeast. No man can safely be allowed to be a judge in his own case.

But there are more complications than this. Thiamine is needed in the diet primarily for the utilization of starch and sugar. A critical factor deciding whether or not a diet is adequately provided with thiamine is, therefore, the proportion of white flour or white rice, and of sugar in it. Of all foods, these are most strikingly lacking in the vitamin; at the same time thiamine is specifically required for their use as sources of energy in the body. The requirement of thiamine by an individual is proportional to the amount of physical work he does, because the more work done, the more calories are needed. At the same time the amount of the vitamin also depends on how much of these calories is derived from dietary components other than fat.

This is part of the background of knowledge upon which estimates have been drawn up of the desirable amounts of a list of different nutrients for an adequate diet. If, after making an assessment of the amounts of nutrients provided by the food which some particular group of the population actually do eat, it is calculated that these are smaller than the official estimate of what they should eat, then the people are listed among those considered to be undernourished.

I think that I have written enough to show that the facts of the matter are such that it is not easy to assert the precise amount of thiamine – using this substance as a single example of a general case – needed in the diet to prevent malnutrition. The signs and symptoms of mild malnutrition are difficult to assess; the nature of the diet itself affects the amount of thiamine needed in it; people vary, and the circumstances in which they live, the amount of exercise they take – all these affect the issue. Because of these real difficulties, it is not surprising that opinions vary. There is little doubt that a starving, emaciated population, some of whom show signs of 'wet' beri-beri, some of 'dry' beri-beri, are rightly categorized as malnourished. But what of a dispirited community, lacking in enterprise, sitting in the shade in Gaza or in a geriatric ward in Manchester or a motel in Florida? In such a group, there may be many whose intake of thiamine is less than the amount that Western dieticians are taught to consider adequate, without any of them showing unequivocal signs of malnutrition.

In such an area of doubt, the best-informed observer must recognize that he is subject to self-interest and self-deception. He has a stock of vitamin tablets to sell; here are customers who could be persuaded to buy; they will get better and he will get richer. It is not the business of the seller to find out whether the lassitude, incompetence and lack of ambition åre due to some cause other than malnutrition. There are in Great Britain, in the United States, and in European countries as well, reputable firms of pharmaceutical manufacturers who circularize industrialists with persuasive literature pointing out – perfectly correctly – that malnutrition affects the physical efficiency and mental alertness of those suffering from it, that industrial accidents are more likely to be caused by those whose health is impaired than by those in full vigour, and that people who do not understand the principles of nutrition may choose an inadequate diet. Often the promotional leaflets continue with more dubious assertions about the connection between dietary deficiency and infection. The upshot of the argument is, that industrialists have a duty to buy multi-vitamin tablets to ensure that their workpeople are kept free from malnutrition and that by doing their duty they will, as an added bonus, profit financially. Who could resist such an argument?

The laws of science are not really laws at all. The facts, measurements and observations upon which science depends may be the sons of heaven, but the deductions drawn from them – useful and fruitful though they may prove to be – are indeed only men's daughters and fallible at that. The textbooks of nutrition may quote the figures for vitamin A which are given in the 'Recommended Dietary Allowances' of the Food and Nutrition Board of the National Academy of Sciences of the United States;[4] or they may prefer the table of the Report of the Committee on Nutrition of the British Medical Association,[5] or half a dozen other all equally reputable authorities. But science does not depend on authority, it depends on thinking. Consider vitamin A.

The eyes of rats – and of children – fed on a diet lacking in vitamin A become dry. This condition of xerophthalmia leads to infection of the cornea of the eye and often progresses to blindness. In less severe deficiency of vitamin A, the natural ability of a man's eye to adapt to seeing in a dim light after having been exposed to bright illumination is lost. To try to discover how much vitamin A is needed to prevent

[4] Food and Nutr. Board, Pub. 302, Nat. Acad. Sci.; Nat. Res. Council, Washington, 1953.
[5] *Rept. Cttee. Nutr.*, BMA, London, 1950.

SELF-DECEPTION AND SELF-INTEREST

either of these harmful effects, the British Medical Research Council[6] organized a heroic experiment in 1949 in which a group of people submitted themselves to a restricted diet for a long time. Even then, however, it was difficult to come to a precise conclusion. Vitamin A-activity is present in different forms in different foods; the presence of other components – fats and the like – affect its efficiency, and it is not easy to know the point at which 'just enough' merges into 'just too little'. The American authorities decided that they would recommend double what they estimated to be the minimum requirement. Part of their argument was that 'there is evidence that dividends in health and more effective physiologic function may accrue when quantities of vitamin A are allowed which are in excess of those required to prevent signs and symptoms of deficiency. By supplying rats from five to ten times the amount of vitamin which prevented deficiency, Sherman and his associates[7] observed that the life span was prolonged, the rate of weight gain increased, and reproduction functions improved'.

The 'recommended dietary allowances' put forward by the Food and Nutrition Board of the US Academy of Science occupy a curious and interesting position midway between science and politics. They are based on the sure and certain touchstone of biochemistry. The vitamin thiamine – all the vitamins indeed and every nutrient as well – possesses an exact and determinable chemical configuration. It performs a precise function in the metabolism of living cells – in those of rats and pigeons as well as in Frenchmen, Congolese and American men and women. The Scots have a saying that when it comes to the final analysis 'we are all Jock Thomson's bairns'. We are all liable to beri-beri, scurvy and pellagra and, without food, we all starve. But the standard table of 'recommended dietary allowances' is not intended to show the 'minimal requirements of nutrients recognized to be necessary for the prevention of nutritional deficiency'. No: they are 'the allowances . . . designed for the maintenance of good nutrition of healthy persons in the United States under present conditions (1953)'.

An American nutritional scientist, brought up as an American to believe that the 'business of the United States is business', that to encourage trade – in motor-cars, oil-paintings or Florida oranges – is

6 Med. Res. Council, *Sp. Rep. Ser.*, 264, London, 1949.
7 Sherman, H. C., and Trupp, H. Y., *Proc. Nat. Acad. Sci.*, 35, 92, 1949.

91

good, and that to consume is even better, will, as a scientist, no matter how hard he struggles to maintain his objectivity, tend to see clearest the evidence that double the amount of vitamin A than is strictly necessary is better than just enough; and that – since Sherman's rats, given five to ten times as much as could be justified on logical grounds, lived longer – Americans *might* live longer if they too ate more.

If the facts which I have tried to gather together in this book prove anything, it is that to assess the human situation and make a right judgement about it is difficult. Experts are valuable people in a complex science-based world. It would be foolish for every man to attempt to be his own radio engineer, motor mechanic and physician. There is, therefore, a place for authority in nutrition. My suggestion now is, however, that the nutritional expert can best apply his special knowledge to understanding, say, the biochemistry of pernicious anaemia and the mechanism of vitamin B_{12}, with its strange cobalt-containing molecule, cobalamin. Or that he can usefully relate the chemistry of protein to his understanding of energy metabolism of the body, and the composition of blood plasma to the symptoms of hunger oedema. In fact, the specialist in nutritional science, as in all other areas of scientific knowledge, is most effective when he applies his knowledge to a restricted field.

Biochemistry and physiology, out of which nutrition developed, can claim, with at least some measure of conviction, to belong to the exact sciences. But the special difficulty of the nutritional scientist is that, when he deals, not with patients under confinement in hospitals, or experimental subjects in laboratories, but with free men and women in the changing and moving communities of the complex world of real life, then he too is only a man as other men are. The nutritionist has at hand a useful tool in his special knowledge, but other men have tools as well – common sense, political experience, financial judgement, administrative ability, knowledge of the history, customs and religion of the peoples with whom they are called upon to deal, kindness, sympathy, yes, and perhaps more *honesty* even than the scientist can claim. Under these circumstances, the nutritional scientist must be an educated man as well as a scientist, and wise too, if he is able; while the citizen can usefully understand the principles of science so that he can test what the nutritionist tells him if he thinks that it ought to be tested. It does not require an unduly profound education to realize that Americans, even if they eat twice as much vitamin A as they need, do not extend their life-span significantly thereby. And while one of the chemical functions of vitamin A is known to be the re-conversion of the retinal pigment, *rhodospin*, which becomes bleached in bright light, to its receptive state as *visual purple*, so that – when vitamin A is seriously lacking from a man's tissues he will suffer from night-blindness (so-called hemeralopia) – it does not necessarily follow that everybody who has difficulty in adapting his eyes to a dim light is suffering from a deficiency of vitamin A. When nutritionists suggest that night-blindness is always due to malnutrition, they may be deceiving themselves as well as their audience. Nutrition is an important scientific topic, but its exponents overestimate their own importance if they bring themselves to believe – as they did in Great Britain during World War II – that their learning can contribute to military success by causing pilots of night-flying aircraft to eat carrots, as a rich source of vitamin-A activity, before taking off on each mission. Many of the scientists who *did* believe this have since learned the bitter lesson that the shrewd advisers of the War Cabinet did *not*, but circulated the rumour that the successes of the R.A.F. were due to carrots, in order to conceal from the enemy the fact that radar was being used.

It should be said that night-blindness, which does indeed result from a shortage of vitamin A, may also be due to a variety of other causes and particularly to heredity. And it must also be said that when there is enough vitamin A in the diet, there is no evidence that more will in any way improve the speed and completeness with which the eyes recover their facility to see in a dim light after having been dazzled by a bright one.

The self-deception of scientists, just like the self-deception of cigarette-manufacturers, is often a group phenomenon. Sincere and honourable cigarette-manufacturers find particular difficulty in accepting the evidence showing that cigarette-smoking is linked with cancer of the lung. Similarly, the distinguished American scientists who drew up the Recommended Dietary Allowances of the US National Academy of Sciences, as well as the numerous groups of students who accepted their authority for the figures, embraced almost as an article of religious faith the estimate 75 mg. as the amount of vitamin C necessary for the wellbeing of a man. The British clung with equal zeal to the figure of 30 mg. Scurvy can, in fact, be cured with 16 mg. or so. Yet British and American scientists became quite hot in arguing their respective cases against each other.

Authority is necessary for an administrator, but it is dangerous for a scientist – particularly so where his science is to be applied under the subtle and complex conditions of a human community inevitably existing in a state of continually shifting flux. Professor Hubbert of Stanford University has argued[8] that to permit authoritarianism into matters of science stultifies progress towards the truth. He also points out that it is unnecessary. The argument that everyone in the modern world – scientists as well as laymen – must accept authoritarianism because of the very immensity of human knowledge, is unsound. Science advances by the unifying generalizations conceived by the few really great scientists. When there are a dozen conflicting explanations of the cause of a condition, and twenty contradictory cures, it can be taken that the proper explanation has still to be reached. When authority writes of 'dividends in health and more effective physiologic function', it is useful for the reader to consider the basic evidence upon which knowledge of the nutritional significance of vitamin A is based.

Before the time of Pasteur, the nature of infectious diseases was quite obscure. One physician would recommend that bedroom windows be kept shut in order to exclude the dangerous night air, another would recommend cold baths, while at one time there was a vogue for electrical treatment.[9] In its day, phlebotomy – the drawing of therapeutic amounts of blood – was as popular a treatment for a variety of illnesses as the administration of castor oil was in the period which came later. The same confusion existed in dietetics before a unifying principle of nutritional science was discovered. This was provided by Hopkins and Mellanby in England, Steenbock in the United States, Jansen in the Netherlands, and many others in the 1920s and 1930s in their experimental studies, by which the existence of vitamins and other so-called 'accessory food factors' became clear and their function known. This knowledge enormously simplified understanding of human and animal physiology and made it possible to design a nutritious diet on a logical basis of knowledge, rather than on opinion and custom.

.   .   .

[8] Hubbert, M. K., *Science* 139, 884, 1963.
[9] Wesley, J., *Primitive Physic*, 1747, Epworth London, 1960.

Not long after World War I, a revolution occurred in the manufacture of cooking utensils. Quite suddenly the manufacturers and traders whose prosperity depended on the trade in iron pots and pans realized that the progress of science and technology was putting them out of business. The new metal, aluminium, unknown to the ancients and only first isolated in metallic form by Hans Christian Oersted in 1825, and then as little more than a laboratory curiosity, became freely available. Compared with iron – and with copper as well – aluminium possessed many advantages. It was lighter, it did not corrode, but above all it conducted heat so much more effectively that the heat of the stove was spread by conductivity over the entire bottom of a pot so that the food in it cooked quicker and with less danger of local overheating. How were the makers of the old pots and pans to stay in business?

'Due to the advent of aluminum cooking utensils', wrote the American journal, *Hygeia*, in 1929, 'the sale of other types of ware for this purpose has been greatly injured. As a result there has been considerable propaganda during the past few years that the cooking of food in aluminum was a common cause of cancer.'

This incident in the history of aluminium serves as a classic example of the way in which people whose actions are ostensibly based on science, which itself is based on fact, come to take up an attitude in which they deceive themselves. Of the principal protagonists of the thesis that aluminium utensils cause cancer, it is perhaps unwise to express an opinion. The beginning of the campaign is usually attributed[10] to a dentist in Toledo, Illinois, Charles T. Betts. This man expressed in the most violent and dogmatic terms his belief that the use of aluminium cooking vessels was a serious menace to public health and unquestionably was a predisposing factor in the spread of cancer in civilized countries.

Talk of angels and you hear their wings. Look for flying saucers and you shall see them. Watch long enough for the Loch Ness monster and it will appear to you. Even in science, as I have written before, experiments are sometimes done to prove a point rather than to obtain information. A scientist who wishes hard enough, can sometimes make his experiments bring his wish to pass. And so, among many others, we find Dr R. M. Le Hunte Cooper

---

[10] 'A Select Annotated Bibliography of the Hygienic Aspects of Aluminum and Aluminum Utensils,' *Mellen Inst. Bull.*, No. 3, 1932.

reporting[11] that aluminium has 'irritative, inflammatory, ulcerative and paretic effects upon the gastric and intestinal mucosa, and apparently seriously damages the nervous system'. These symptoms were improved in certain cases, which he quoted, when the use of aluminium cooking utensils was discontinued.

Dr Cooper was just one of an evanescent host who, first for one reason then for another, deceive themselves. Wisdom is for each generation equally difficult to attain, and the short history of modern science has already shown that scientists, and particularly those concerned with food, can never assume their immunity from self-deception. In a solid review article, Blumenthal[12] referred to world-wide propaganda against aluminium cooking vessels. Whether or not its origin was plain dishonesty by the makers of iron vessels, sincere and worthy men believed it and found evidence to support their belief. Besides Dr Cooper there was Dr Francis[13] who cited six cases of patients who gave up the use of aluminium vessels and thereby were freed from abdominal pain.

Were it not for the wideness with which this extraordinary belief in the unwholesomeness of food cooked in aluminium was held, it would not be worth referring to the matter now at a time when aluminium foil, aluminium saucepans, indeed aluminium vessels and equipment of all sorts are accepted as a matter of course. But, as I shall show, because people who believe their outlook is scientific have deceived themselves in the past is no insurance that their successors will not do the same in the future. And deception once started is slow and hard to stop. To put an end to the unfounded fears about aluminium needed a report by the German Federal Health Department,[14] a review in a French journal,[15] an extensive study by the Mellen Institute in America,[16] and a report by the director of the Pharmaceutical Society of Great Britain.[17]

But scientists, even with all this power that knowledge brings, still remain men whose judgement power may insidiously corrupt. A

[11] Cooper, R. M. Le H., *Brit. Med. J.,* 26 Mar. 1932.
[12] Blumenthal, C., *German J. Cancer Res.,* 30 Heft 3, 1929.
[13] Francis, A., *Brit. Med. J.,* 16 Apr. 1932.
[14] Blumenthal, C., *German J. Cancer Res.,* 30, Heft 3, 1929.
[15] Ichok J., *Ann. Hyg.,* 1929.
[16] 'A Select Annotated Bibliography of the Hygienic Aspects of Aluminum and Aluminum Utensils,' *Mellen Inst. Bull.,* No. 3, 1932.
[17] Barn, J. H., *Brit. Med. J.,* 11 Jun. 1932.

powerful king – even an intelligent one – cannot bear to think that his power is limited, so sometimes he believes that what his courtiers say is true. The power of thiamine to cure beri-beri and of niacin to cure pellagra, implies that vitamin E, for lack of which female rats reabsorb their unborn young, must be a powerful agent too. At one time, so convinced were certain workers[18] in its efficiency in treating heart disease that over twenty thousand Canadian patients were treated with it. Yet the evidence implies that this belief was misplaced.

The history of science is littered with examples of furious controversy. Where it would be imagined that an ice-cold researcher would assess the evidence and, solely on this evidence, reach a tentative conclusion, it is, in fact, often found that, having accepted an idea – from a teacher or often from a persuasive pharmaceutical advertisement – the alleged scientist holds to it with fervour. It would almost appear that he takes active steps to deceive himself. If this is so with scientists, how can he blame chocolate-bar manufacturers from bringing themselves to believe that the confectionery they sell – even though the most expensive source of calories, even though it satiates the children who eat it and spoils their appetite for more nutritious food, and even though there is good evidence to show that in the communities that can afford chocolates and sweets obesity among children is a more serious problem than nutritional deficiency – even though all this is known, how can the scientists blame the manufacturers for coming actually to believe that by disseminating their products they are doing the children good and giving them 'energy'?

Self-deception, even when it is not aggravated by self-interest, is hard to avoid. It is sometimes equally difficult to diagnose or discover the reason why, presented with the same set of facts, one man will reach – and afterwards firmly hold – one point of view while another will insist on a different conclusion.

In 1953 Dr Ancel Keys,[19] working in Minneapolis, drew attention to the fact that communities in which the incidence of coronary heart disease was high ate a diet containing a large proportion of fat. Before long it was observed that better correlation was between the

[18] Shute, W. E. and Shute, E. V., 'Vitamin E', Natural Vitamin Foundation, N.Y., 1940–60.
[19] Keys, A., *J. Mnt. Sinai Hosp.*, 20, 118, 1953.

incidence of the disease and the consumption of fats, such as butter, lard and mutton fat, in which the proportion of 'saturated' fatty acids was particularly high. Later on, it was concluded that it was not only the amount of such fat that a man ate which affected the likelihood of his suffering from so-called ischaemic heart disease, but also the degree to which he failed to take physical exercise. Eventually, the relative proportion of saturated and unsaturated fatty acids, the total amount of fat in the diet, the amount of sugar in the diet, the level of cholesterol in the bloodstream, the presence or absence of obesity, and the amount of exercise taken were all suspected of playing a part. In 1966, the situation was summarized by the American Medical Association thus: 'Does dietary fat relate to coronary artery disease? Despite vast researches conducted since World War II, the answers are not unanimous. Clinicopathologic, biochemical, experimental, and epidemiologic data, gathered in many lands, lend themselves to conflicting interpretations'.[20]

We have here a current problem the solution of which is – as is so much in real life – by no means clear. Like the manufacturers of chocolate-bars and cigarettes, we all have an 'interest' in the outcome. People who like good living, mutton chops and plenty of butter and cream, will wish that there is no truth in the hypothesis that such foods tend to induce heart disease. Farmers and provision merchants will hope so too. On the other hand, people marketing cooking oil containing a high proportion of unsaturated fatty acid, and those spiritually and intellectually committed to the hypothesis that fat is concerned with coronary disease, will be predisposed to believe any supporting evidence. Two historical studies illustrate my theme.

Believing that it is easier to reach a cool judgement by standing a little back from the subject, Dr L. Michaels[21] studied the census records of England and Wales of the eighteenth and nineteenth centuries. He collected details of the causes of death of some millions of middle-aged men of the middle and upper social classes. These are the principal candidates for coronary heart disease today. According to such information as is available, the diet of these men one or two hundred years ago was as rich and ample as is that of their successors today, perhaps more so. And nobody was reported as dying of coronary heart disease. Indeed, the very first description of angina

[20] Editorial, *J. Amer. Med. Ass.*, 197, 723, 1966.
[21] Michaels, L., *Brit. Heart J.*, 28, 258, 1966.

pectoris was in 1768, the first account of coronary thrombosis was in 1880 and the first account of myocardial infarction appeared in 1912. Michaels considers it inconceivable that if these conditions had in fact occurred, the great physicians of earlier times, Galen, Paracelsus or Sydenham, who accurately described such diseases as gout or migraine, could possibly have failed to report such comparatively dramatic conditions as angina pectoris and coronary thrombosis. In the light of this conviction, the paradox of the virtual absence of any accounts at all of these diseases, despite the consumption of diets rich in fat and frequent reference to the sin of gluttony – equated in turpitude at that time with lechery – led Michaels to conclude that, whatever else it may be due to, the alarming rise of heart disease as the twentieth-century killer of middle-aged men cannot be due to dietary fats.

Is Michaels right in his interpretation or – like a driver involved in a traffic accident who can never conceive of himself as being its cause – is he the victim of self-deception?

At about the same time that Michaels published his historical study of England and Wales, another investigator, H. B. Sprague,[22] reviewed the situation as it had existed in the United States and reached the diametrically opposite conclusion on the past incidence of coronary artery disease. In his view, early vital statistics should be approached critically and with considerable scepticism. He argued that coronary deaths had appeared in the records listed as 'apoplexy', 'sudden death' or 'dropsy'. His conclusion was that: 'Certainly, the disease did not suddenly leap into existence about 1920, fully armed for destruction like Athena from the brow of Zeus.' Considering the same situation as that reviewed by Michaels, the one on one side of the Atlantic, the other on the other, Sprague concluded that there was no significant difference in the prevalence of coronary artery disease beyond that expected from population growth, and that – there being little change in the estimated amount of dietary fat – the past presented no striking contrast with the present. In fact, Sprague considered that the evidence of the past, like that of the present, supported the hypothesis that dietary fat *is* concerned with heart disease.

The moral for the student of nutritional science is clear. In the words of Oliver Cromwell to the General Assembly of the Church of

[22] Sprague, H. B., *Arch. Environ. Health*, 13, 4, 1966.

Scotland: 'I beseech you, in the bowels of Christ, think it possible you may be mistaken.' God's sons are indeed things. These things, the facts and observations of nature, are the groundwork of science. Maintain a patient on a diet containing a calculated quantity of saturated fat and, as the amount of fat is increased, the level of cholesterol in his blood will rise. This is fact. But its interpretation is more difficult. Keys' original statistics were very convincing: he showed that in countries where the amount of saturated fats consumed was large (the United States, Finland, Scotland) the proportion of men between 45 and 49 dying of heart disease was high – 251, 220 and 189 per 100,000 in 1957–8;[23] whereas in countries where the consumption of such fats was less (Sweden, France, Japan) the death from this cause was also less frequent – 69, 38 and 44 per 100,000. Then, when closer scrutiny was made, other factors, some of which I have mentioned, also seemed to play a part. There is even a plausible relationship between statistics for deaths from coronary heart disease and the number of television sets in the community!

This brings me to one more dangerous self-deception to which the modern food scientist is particularly liable. It is the belief that the pursuit of nutrition is the cardinal goal of man on earth and the target of civilization. 'An over-all program of nutrition education must,' wrote L. A. Maynard[24], 'do more than teach the individual good eating habits. It should also develop a public consciousness of the importance of good nutrition and of sound food policies for the promotion of our national vigour and stability. Ill-fed people do not make good citizens. Employers need a greater appreciation of how good nutrition increases work efficiency and cuts down absenteeism. Taxpayers need to realize that good nutrition decreases public expenditures for medical care and for the support of those unable to earn their own living.'

We live in a period of history when science has become accepted as the principal underlying philosophy of our society. If a man is unhappy he turns to scientific medicine for relief: no one in a twentieth-century community would seek advice from a hermit or a wise man. But science owes its phenomenal success to the fact that its exponents restrict their attack to a narrow front. Progress is unlikely when the target of attack is the cure for cancer, it is better to study the

[23] WHO, *Epidem. vit. Stat. Rep.*, 15, 89, 1962.
[24] Maynard, L. A., *Nutrition Rev.*, 9, 354, 1951.

mechanisms of cell-division in the epethelial tissues of the mouse. The treatment of pernicious anaemia became really effective only when a few milligrams of vitamin B_{12} had been isolated and the nature of its complex molecule established by a combination of advanced organic chemistry and X-ray crystallography.

A physician must do the best he can for his patient whether or not the nature of pernicious anaemia, cancer or the common cold has been worked out. That is why the practice of medicine is only partly science; the rest is art. For the same reason, the science of nutrition can only partly solve the problems of a community crying for bread. Professor Maynard was a good scientist and a sincere, big-hearted man anxious to serve his generation. But surely he and other nutritionists who have succeeded him deceive themselves if they believe that it is the 'over-all program of nutrition education' that makes a nation vigorous and stable. Nutrition and the food supply had little to do with the instability of England in the reign of Charles I. Nor is it, indeed, particularly the business of nutritionists in teaching good food habits to use the argument that their teaching should be accepted because it will cut down industrial absenteeism. It may not even be good science; coalminers have been known to take a day off, not because they are hungry but, on the contrary, because they have earned enough to enable them to sacrifice their bonus to prune the roses in their garden.

CHAPTER VIII

IF IT'S POISONOUS, WHY EAT IT?

Anyone introducing a new food into a modern industrialized community possessing an efficient and scientifically sophisticated public health system, or developing a new chemical colouring-matter or emulsifier or anti-staling agent, is required to submit it first to prolonged tests on rats and dogs and hamsters and chickens. To satisfy the Food and Drugs Authorities and the Food Standards and Labelling Committee, these tests would occupy a period of years and would cost perhaps £50,000. The tests are in fact so stringent that if Sir Walter Raleigh turned up *now* with the potato, as a new and unknown food, he would never stand a chance of having it accepted. Potatoes contain a poisonous substance, solanine. Wholesome potato tubers contain about 90 parts of solanine per million. This concentration may fairly readily increase if, for example, dug potatoes are exposed for long to the sun. Potatoes containing 400 parts per million have been associated with outbreaks of poisoning.[1]

It is a remarkable social paradox that educated nations accept quite calmly the daily use of a foodstuff commonly containing a toxic agent, of which five times more would prove harmful. As I shall describe later, it is usual to insist on at least a hundredfold margin of safety for anything new. The main reason why it is, in fact, very uncommon for anyone to be poisoned by eating potatoes is because the solanine is mainly concentrated in the sprouts or in the green patches on potatoes which have been exposed unduly long to light. Furthermore, a major proportion of the solanine present in potato tubers is extracted by the cooking water when they are boiled. Cases of poisoning do occur from time to time, however, and have been described in the scientific literature.[2]

The wide use of potatoes, and the extreme rarity of harm arising from their consumption, show that there is little cause for alarm in the knowledge that they contain a toxic agent. The point of interest is

---

[1] Bamford, F., *Poison: their isolation and identification*, Blackiston, Philadelphia, 3rd ed. 1961.

[2] Hansen, A. J. M., *Science*, 61, 340, 1925., Harris, F. W., & Cockburn, F., *Am. J. Pharm.*, 90, 722, 1918.

more philosophical than of clinical moment. It is none the less worthy of attention by nutritionists and those concerned with the community's food. Is it not strange that, now that attacks on the potato on religious and magical grounds have died down for two hundred years or more, no breath of protest has been raised by analytical chemists, pharmacologists, national or international public-health authorities, or even food faddists? Yet here is a food which demonstrably contains a toxic material and which *might* contain enough of it to do harm. Nutritionists know how difficult it is to determine precisely how much of each different nutrient needed by the body must be present in the daily food to prevent malnutrition. We have also seen how confusing are the decisions which must be taken in weighing the relative importance of nutritional health on the one hand compared with all the other human motives – self-denial, for example, or social intercourse. Clearly, if the assessment of the positive nutritive constituents of the diet is a problem worthy of consideration, it is equally important to establish a policy by which to judge what is the tolerable level of harmful and toxic components of the foodstuffs of which the diet is made up.

One of the reasons for the popularity of 'escapist' adventure stories and cowboy films is that the values they reflect are simple and direct. The 'goodies' are good and the 'baddies' are bad. Popular publications on nutrition sometimes employ the same approach. There are 'goody' nutritious foods such as green vegetables and milk on the one hand; on the other hand, there are 'chemicals' in food – dyes and preservatives and anti-oxidants – which are 'bad'. The truth, in nutrition as in the narrative of real life, is more complicated. Potatoes are not alone in containing potentially dangerous ingredients.

In 1928, workers at Johns Hopkins Hospital in America[3] happened to notice that a number of the rabbits kept in their laboratory had developed goitre. These rabbits were fed mainly on cabbage. Sir Charles Hercus and his colleagues in New Zealand[4] were struck by this observation and looked into the matter more closely. They found that not only cabbage, but turnips too, and particularly the *seeds* of cabbage, mustard and rape contained a toxic material that caused goitre.

[3] Chesney, A. M., Clawson, T. A., & Webster, B., *Bull, John. Hopk. Hosp.* 43, 261, 1928.
[4] Hercus, C. E., and Purues, H.D., *J. Hyg. Camb,* 36, 182, 19 36.

As a matter of fact the goitre-producing substance, 1-5-vinyl-2-thio-oxazolidene, is quite widespread among the green vegetables which are particularly recommended by dieticians for their wholesomeness. It has been isolated from kale, brussels-sprouts, broccoli, rape and kohlrabi as well as cabbage.[5]

Goitre is a disease commonly caused by a deficiency of iodine in the diet. In order to function properly, the thyroid gland in the neck needs to accumulate a sufficiency of iodine. The harmful effect of oxazolidene is due to the fact that it prevents this accumulation. In parts of the world where the local foodstuffs are deficient in iodine, cabbage can exert a toxic effect when it is eaten directly or, as it were, at second hand. For example, in 1955, the incidence of goitre among children in Tasmania was increasing in spite of the use of iodized salt. It appeared that the farmers, anxious to increase supplies of milk, were feeding their expanding herds of dairy cows on 'many-headed kale'. It was eventually concluded[6] that the oxazolidene from the kale was being absorbed by the cows in sufficient concentration to contaminate their milk.

Anyone attempting to reach a balanced judgement of the two aspects of cabbage – the positive contribution of vitamin C and vitamin A-activity, and the negative content of goitreogenic toxicity – might usefully bear in mind the following curious appendix. Having observed the way in which the supply of iodine to the thyroid was blocked by the eating of cabbage, Astwood[7] – thinking that it might contain thiourea, a substance known to produce this effect – tried administering thiourea to patients suffering from the condition of hyperthyroidism caused by an overactive thyroid. This was so successful that it became the basis of modern medical treatment of this disease.

And then there is rhubarb. Generations of children, not much liking it, have been compelled to eat up this vegetable masquerading as a fruit 'to do them good'. Yet it may contain significant amounts of the salts of oxalic acid, an organic acid which is toxic to both man and livestock. An essential physiological prerequisite for health is that the concentration of mineral ions in the bloodstream should

[5] Nordfelt, S., Gellerstadt, N., and Falkmer, S., *Act. Path. Microbiol. Scand.*, 35, 217, 1954.
[6] Clements, F. W., *Med. J. Aust.*, 2, 369, 1955.
[7] Astwood, E. B., *J. Pharmacol.*, 78, 79, 1943.

remain constant. Absorption of oxalate tends to cause the proper concentration of calcium to fall. In one study of sheep which died after eating rhubarb it was found that the concentration of calcium in their blood was only one-fifth of the normal value at the time of their death.[8] The symptoms of this oxalate poisoning were reduced coagulability of the blood, acute nephritis, and nervous effects as well.

The leaves of rhubarb contain more oxalate than the stalks, which are most commonly eaten. Yet under certain circumstances even the lower concentrations have been shown to be potentially harmful. Kohman;[9] for example, fed spinach – another food popular for its vitamin content, but also containing oxalate – for a prolonged period to experimental laboratory animals which were receiving a diet low in calcium, and found that it was fatal. When people eat the more highly toxic parts of the rhubarb plant, they suffer. During World War I when the more conventional kinds of vegetables became scarce in Great Britain, the population were officially recommended to eat rhubarb leaves. As a result, several cases of fatal poisoning occurred.[10] A more remarkable case was reported at about the same time from Montana where a woman who ate a meal of fried rhubarb leaves died within thirty-six hours.[11]

It might be argued, although the argument is a weak one, that as rhubarb is a common and familiar food, it is not surprising if its potential toxicity is overlooked or, if not overlooked, forgiven. Avocados, on the other hand, are a delicacy. By what right or logic, therefore, have they escaped pharmacological scrutiny? Not only have instances of poisoning been reported among cattle, horses, goats, rabbits, canaries and fish after having eaten them;[12] but, when they were submitted to test in the laboratory, the fruit[13] and the leaves as well[14] were found to contain a toxic substance. The effect on animals may be serious. Cows, goats and mares develop acute mastitis. Goats may be so severely poisoned that they die. Rabbits

---

[8] Vawter, L. R., *California Vet.*, 31, 12, 1950.

[9] Kohman, E. F., *J. Nutrition*, 18, 233, 1939.

[10] Anon., *Sci. Amer.*, 117, 82, 1917.

[11] Robb, H. F., *J. Amer. Med. Ass.*, 73, 627, 1919.

[12] Hurt, L., *Ann. Rep. Los Angeles County Livestock Dept.*, 44, 1942–3.

[13] Valeri, H., and Gimeno, N., *Rev. de. Med. Vet. y Parasit.* (Caracas) 12, 131, 1953.

[14] Appleman, D., *California Avocado Soc. Yearbook*, 37, 1944.

fed on the leaves of one particular variety died within twenty-four hours although they were unaffected by leaves from a different variety. Clearly some kinds of avocado may contain more of the toxic agent than others. A curious case reported by Professor Kingsbury[15] was that of canaries fed on ripe avocado pears being poisoned. Although avocados do not as a general rule form a major part of human diets, nevertheless it is perhaps paradoxical that such an exotic food should have escaped scrutiny by nutritionists although the canary, used as a sensitive detector of air unfit for men in coalmines and submarines, has proved to be susceptible also to this new danger.

Onions, like potatoes and cabbages, are common articles of diet. But whereas potatoes and cabbages are recommended by scientific experts as vehicles for vitamin C (obtainable for the most part only from fruit and vegetables) and for other nutritional advantages, onion does not possess much in the way of nutritional virtues. It is, however, popular for its characteristic taste and smell. This absence of demonstrable nutritional value has been found puzzling by a number of investigators. Folk-lore has attributed a number of qualities to onion: it has been alleged to prevent rheumatism, to cure colds, and to be a generally health-giving food. In terms of its chemical composition it is not impressive; but scientists have, nevertheless, borne in mind that traditional folk-beliefs have from time to time been found to be correct. In 1930, Dr Henry Sebrell[16] carried out a study to discover whether onions contained a particular vitamin of the 'B$_2$-group' which was at that time being investigated as a possible agent for the cure of the disease pellegra. To his surprise, he discovered that, far from contributing vitamin activity to the diet, the addition of either raw or cooked onions to the dogs' ration caused severe anaemia. It has since been found that dogs are not alone in their susceptibility to whatever may be the toxic agent in onions. Horses have also been poisoned.[17] Within about a week of having been given access to a quantity of onions, horses and cattle developed anaemia and a number of other symptoms from which some of them died, particularly if they were forced into sudden activity. Curiously enough,

[15] Kingsbury, J. R., *Poisonous Plants of the United States and Canada*, Prentice Hall, 1964.
[16] Sebrell, W. H., *US Pub. Health Rep.*, 24, 1175, 1930.
[17] Thorp, F., and Harshfield, G. S., *J. Amer. Vet. Med. Assoc.*, 94, 52, 1939.

older animals are often more seriously affected than the younger ones. Again it seems curious and paradoxical, in view of the attention with which nutritionists have studied some of the components of food – protein and vitamins, for example – that no attention has been paid to so striking a property of so common an article. If people are as susceptible to onion-poisoning as dogs, they would need to eat only about three-quarters of a pound a day fairly regularly to give themselves anaemia. Although there may not be many people who do eat this amount of onions, the margin of safety is much less than that for other components of food about which alarms have been expressed. I shall discuss some of these later on.

Perhaps the strong burning taste of horseradish saves us from doing ourselves a mischief by eating it, just as the transient vertigo experienced when smoking a strong cigar warns the smoker to desist before he injures himself. Mustard oil, the poisonous principle in horseradish,[18] contains a mixture of allyl-iso-thiocyanate and beta-phenyl-iso-thiocyanate. The amount of horseradish which in three hours killed a pig which ate it was of the order of 1 lb. – a quantity which few normal people would ever eat. Nevertheless, here is an example of another article of food which is patently poisonous – cattle and horses have died, as well as pigs, from eating both tops and roots[19] – a fact to which no public attention is paid.

For those who try to clear their minds on how best to decide what is poisonous and what is not, broad beans provide a particularly puzzling problem. The scientific literature is full of references to peculiar poisonings by broad beans, and not mainly of animals, but of people. Broad beans, native to the Mediterranean region where they are widely cultivated, have throughout history been used as food for men and animals. Yet some people who eat them, especially if they eat them raw or partly cooked, may develop acute hepatitis. Even though only certain people are susceptible, toxic reaction is so well recognized that it ranks as a disease under the name of 'favism', the botanical name for broad beans being *Vicia faba*. This disease is common among Sardinians, although it occurs in other Mediterranean areas as well. Only people of certain race, family and sex – males are more commonly affected than females – seem to contract favism. For example, it may afflict Americans of Italian or Jewish

[18] Forsyth, A. A., Min. of Ag., Fish. and Food, London, *Bull.* 161, 1954.
[19] Hackett, W., *J. Comp. Path. and Therapeut.*, 30, 138, 1917.

parentage. The disease may be serious, and about one in ten of children who contract it die.[20]

Not only may broad beans prove poisonous when they are eaten, but symptoms of favism may occur within minutes of bean pollen being inhaled. When broad beans are eaten by a susceptible individual, headache, dizziness, nausea, vomiting and a raised temperature may occur within 5 to 24 hours. In more severe cases, haemolytic anaemia and collapse may follow.

The interesting feature of this whole business is that it is now clear[21] that victims of favism possess an inherited abnormality of their red blood cells which are deficient in a particular enzyme, glucose-6-phosphate-dehydrogenase. In this instance, therefore, we have a food, commonly accepted as a wholesome vegetable, yet one which is highly toxic, indeed sometimes lethal, to one particular, genetically-segregated group of the human population.

A different kind of danger which may be in wait for one special category of people from a common food, is presented by cheese: particularly Cheddar cheese. The people at risk this time are not a genetically-linked group of Sardinians or American Jews. The danger instead hangs over patients suffering from depression who have been prescribed by their doctors a group of drugs which inhibit the enzyme mono-amine-oxidase. These drugs, of which *isoniazid* is perhaps the best known, have been particularly effective, and are quite widely used. In 1955, Ogilvie[22] observed that some patients taking isoniazid were suddenly afflicted with attacks of severe headache associated with palpitations, flushes, sweats and raised blood pressure. The cause of these alarming incidents remained unknown for eight years until, in 1963, Blackwell and Womack[23] found that they were caused by eating cheese. The toxic component in the cheese was identified as tyramine.[24] Normally, people eating cheese can break down any tyramine in it into a harmless compound which is subsequently excreted from the body. Patients taking mono-amine-oxidase-inhibiting drugs, however, are unable to carry out this detoxicating operation in their tissues, and suffer accordingly.

[20] Luisada, A., *Medicine, 20,* 229, 1941.
[21] Linkham, W. H., Lenhard, R. E., and Childs, *B. J. Plasm. and Exp. Therapeut.,* 122, 85A, 1958.
[22] Ogilvie, C. M., *Quart. J. Med.,* 24, 175, 1955.
[23] Blackwell, B., and Womack, A. M., *Lancet,* II, 414, 463, 1963.
[24] Asatoor, A. M., Levi, A. J., and Milne, M. D., *Lancet,* II, 733, 1963.

The problem for the nutritionist concerned with food safety is quite a subtle one. Not all cheeses are equally toxic. Cheddar cheese has most frequently been incriminated; but, again, only some Cheddar cheeses are harmful. In fact, the amount of tyramine in different samples has been found to vary from 0 to 953 parts per million.[25] It seems that when the cheese is made, the bacterial culture used to curdle the milk and give the finished product its flavour may contain a mixture of organisms some of which produce tyramine while others do not. In this instance, therefore, we have a manufacturing process of great antiquity in which, unknown to the manufacturer, a substance of high pharmacological activity and potential toxicity – tyramine – is produced in fluctuating amounts.

It is, perhaps, a different matter for a nutritionist to be on his guard against the sort of poison which poisons everybody – like solanine in potatoes, goitreogenic agents in cabbage, and anaemia-producing toxins in onions – and, on the other hand, compounds such as tyramine which can be expected only to harm those people who are taking a particular kind of drug. Nevertheless the latter category of substances is quite diverse. The fact that a food may not harm everybody who eats it is no justification for the responsible man to overlook the possibility that it may poison somebody. An interesting example is provided by strawberries.

Coumarin is an aromatic organic compound which occurs in a number of plant species. It possesses an agreeable and characteristic smell, and a pleasant taste. Because it was known to be a natural component of several kinds of food articles, and also because of its attractive taste and smell, it was not long ago proposed to use it as a flavouring agent. It is true that, when large amounts of coumarin are eaten, it interferes with the clotting of the blood, and may in consequence give rise to uncontrollable bleeding following what would otherwise have been trivial injury. It was considered, however, that the amounts needed as a flavouring agent were so much less than those likely to affect the blood's clotting mechanism, that no possible harm could result from its use in food. This argument may be valid for normal people. Are they therefore justified in increasing their happiness by enjoying the enhanced flavour and aroma that coumarin would bring them? The current answer to this philosophical question is *No*. Not because of the minuscule risk to normal people, but

[25] Blackwell, B., and Mabbitt, *Lancet*, I, 938, 1965.

because each year several thousand patients who have recovered from a coronary thrombosis are given for long periods measured doses of coumarin or of a drug which, like coumarin, holds back the clotting of their blood. Should such people eat food flavoured with coumarin, the additional amount could cause haemorrhage.[26]

But the danger for these people is not only from food artificially flavoured in this way. For them foods in which coumarin is a natural constituent – of which strawberries are one – could also be poisonous.

In 1954, a biologist called Paget[27] described a disease which he had observed in his experimental guinea pigs. The symptoms were oedema – which might be described as dropsy – together with a disorder of the liver. This disease, which was not infectious, he called *exudative hepatitis*. After it had been described by Paget, it was observed sporadically in other laboratories, and was always associated with the feeding of a particular pelleted diet containing 15 per cent of groundnut meal. But only certain batches of diet were involved.

Then, in 1957, a number of guinea pigs in a breeding colony at the Central Veterinary Laboratory at Weybridge in Surrey died, and others had abortions. This condition was eventually connected with the presence of toxic groundnut in the diet.[28]

The narrative now changes from a scientific curiosity to a matter of practical importance. In 1960 what seemed to be a new disease caused the death of an estimated 100,000 young turkeys in the turkey-farms of England. The cause of the illness was not known. Soon the same disease began to kill ducklings and young pheasants as well. The following year it was found that the death of the turkeys, ducklings and pheasants alike was due to the incorporation of groundnuts in their rations. These nuts all came from Brazil.[29] Although search was made for a toxic component, its nature at first remained a mystery. The problem became even more confused when the death of ducks on a number of farms in Kenya was found to be due to their having been fed on groundnuts grown and processed, not in Brazil, but in East Africa.

[26] Keckwick, R. T., *J. Mat. Food. Sci. Fed.*, I, 1p, 1966.
[27] Paget, G. E., *J. Path. Bact.*, 67, 393, 1954.
[28] Paterson, J. S., Crook, J. C., Shand, A., Lewis G., & Allcroft, R., *Vet. Rec.*, 74, 639, 1962.
[29] Blount, W. P., *Turkeys*, 9, 52, 1961; Asplin, F. D., & Carnaghan, R. B. A., *Vet. Rec.*, 73, 1215, 1961.

In 1961 and 1962 the hunt was up and hundreds of samples of groundnut meal were tested for toxicity. Occasional poisonous meals were found from groundnuts grown in 13 producing countries in different parts of the world. It was then observed that other species than poultry and guinea pigs were susceptible. Young pigs of 3 to 12 weeks of age were readily affected by the poisonous groundnut meals. So were pregnant sows. Calves from 1 to 6 months old were highly susceptible, and an outbreak of poisoning was found among store cattle in the field.[30] Four-year-old heifers were poisoned by a ration containing 20 per cent of the affected groundnut meal. Ten-year-old cows were not noticeably harmed, although their yield of milk was reduced.

At the best of times, to comprehend food science a level head is required. What then is to be made of the sudden appearance of poisonous groundnuts? The widespread distribution of toxic material and its sporadic appearance led Austwick[31] to the conclusion that the source of the poison was a fungus, later identified[32] as *Aspergillus flavus*, with which the groundnuts had become contaminated. Here then we have the nutritious groundnut, itself a rich source of protein and fat contributing B-vitamins as well, yet the possible vehicle for a poison, now called *aflatoxin*, produced by a fungus which – if conditions during the harvesting, drying and storage of the nuts are warm and humid – chooses to grow on them.

In the comparatively short time since aflatoxin was identified, chemists have been studying its chemistry and have discovered that it may exist in more than one molecular form. Chemical tests on aflatoxin have been developed, and biological methods worked out to measure its toxicity. It is now recognized that contaminated feeds and foodstuffs may not only be highly toxic, but are carcinogenic as well. In rats, the isolated aflatoxin has been found to be the most active substance known for producing cancer of the liver.[33] Mice, on the other hand, appear to be quite immune.[34] An odd phenomenon of a growing incidence of liver cancers among hatchery-reared rainbow

---

[30] Clegg, F. G., & Bryson, H., *Vet. Rec.*, 74, 992, 1962.
[31] Austwick, P. K. C., quoted by Carnaghan, R. B. A., & Allcroft, R., *Chem. & Ind.*, 881, 53, 1963.
[32] Sargeant, K., Sheridan, A., O'Kelly, J., & Carnaghan, R.B.A. *Nature* 193, 1096, 1961.
[33] Butter, W. H., & Barnes, J. M., *Brit. J. Cancer*, 17, 699, 1963.
[34] Platonow, N., *Vet. Rec.*, 76, 589, 1964.

trout is now thought to be explained as being due to poisoning by aflatoxin.

And what of ourselves? Is man affected by mould on groundnuts? Has there all along been an element of risk in eating groundnuts, using them for oil for the manufacture of margarine, using them to make peanut butter, or eating meat and drinking milk from poultry and cattle fed on them? The answer may be yes.

Primary liver cancers are particularly prevalent among the inhabitants of certain parts of Africa and Asia. Mouldy maize and groundnuts are important ingredients of many African diets, and it is by no means improbable that the high incidence of liver tumours in young adult Bantus and Senegalese[35] may be related to this fact. And aflatoxin may not be alone. Now that this poisonous compound produced by one type of mould, namely *A. flavus*, has been identified, it is beginning to be suspected that there may be others.[36] Positive proof that these cancers in man, and other ill-effects similar to those seen in animals and birds, are actually due to a toxin in groundnuts is still lacking, but the circumstantial evidence is strong. It is certainly strong enough to encourage the producers and processors of groundnuts to take quite stringent precautions to ensure that groundnuts and groundnut-meal shall not become mouldy, and for public health authorities to analyse samples to ensure the absence of aflatoxin. And for the philosophical student of dietetics here is yet another example of a food, accepted as a commonplace staple of quite significant nutritional quality, originating in South America and spreading from thence to be cultivated in all the tropical and sub-tropical countries of the world, being found to be a potential source of poison.

The lesson of the groundnut toxin is a simple but important one. It is, that this is a dangerous world. Knowledge can teach us to be prudent; but wisdom and experience teach us that in life, whether or not we accept the risk, we can never be absolutely safe. We can only learn, while living dangerously, to behave rationally with as full a knowledge of what we are doing as we can command. Consider, for example, the curious observations of Dr Karel Shama.[37]

Dr Shama, a distinguished entomologist, carried out a series of

[35] Richir *et al., Cent. rend. Seance. Soc. Biol.*, 158, 1375, 1964.
[36] Tatsouno, *Fd. Cosmet. Toxic, 2*, 678, 1964.
[37] Shama, K., & Williams, C. M., *Proc. Nat. Acad, Sci.*, USA, 54, 411, 1965.

112

studies in Prague of the bug, *Pyrrhocoris afertus*. His investigation occupied a period of ten years. At the end of this time, he accepted an engagement in America and, on moving to Boston, took with him his stock of bugs. There, to his mortification, they all unexpectedly died. Because their death was associated with a failure to undergo a normal metamorphosis, Dr Shama concluded that they had been affected by some unknown source of 'juvenile hormone'. It is known that the active principle of this hormone, which prevents metamorphosis, and in the absence of which metamorphosis takes place, is the substance, chemically classified as an alcohol, called farnesol. The cause of the disaster by which Dr Shama's bugs had been overwhelmed was eventually found in truth to be farnesol – with which, it was discovered, the paper towels used in the rearing-jars in which the bugs were confined were contaminated. When the source of this contamination was investigated it was found that, while American paper contained traces of 'juvenile hormone', papers from Europe and Japan did not; bugs kept in contact with paper from the two latter sources throve.

The research was taken deeper. It now appeared that the anti-metamorphosis activity of the American paper was derived from the species of American balsam fir, *Abies balsamea*, from the pulp of which the paper was manufactured. Although in this incident, the non-intentional additive present in American paper affected the health and wellbeing of bugs, there is a moral here for food technologists. This curious biochemical happening serves as a warning that even so apparently innocuous a substance as paper may prove to be a vehicle for pharmacologically active agents; and, furthermore, that significant variations may occur in the composition and in the safety of different batches of paper.

And fir trees, from which paper is made, are not alone in containing physiologically active compounds. Indeed, there are many more striking examples. Since the days of Pliny and Dioscorides the beautiful green oleander, with its showy pink and white blossom, has been recognized to be a poisonous plant. It contains at least two highly poisonous principles which possess a pharmacological activity somewhat similar to digitalis. The medical literature is full of stories of men and animals dying after eating only tiny quantities of the leaves.[38]

[38] Steyn, D. G., *The toxicology of plants in South Africa*, Johannesburg, 1934.

113

As recently as 1957, there was a report[39] of a number of people being severely poisoned after eating frankfurters which had been roasted over a fire made of sticks from an oleander tree. Other accounts have appeared of soldiers dying of poisoning after roasting meat skewered on oleander sticks. Horses too have been killed after being tethered, and only for a very short time, to oleander bushes.

This is all unquestionably very alarming. Yet the reason why we can be calm in the knowledge that hydrangeas contain cyanogenic glycosides, and that the *Journal of the American Medical Association* described the painful symptoms suffered by a horse which ate a potted hydrangea;[40] that rhododendrons contain a toxic ingredient which has been isolated but not yet identified; and even that oleander is among the most poisonous plants known is, that we accept the hazards of the world and the need for prudent behaviour. Just as we know that smoking cigarettes is so dangerous a practice that sensible people must – if they smoke at all – do it judiciously and with temperate balance, so also are we prepared to face the risks inherent in eating horseradish, onions, potatoes, cabbages and broad beans. The foods which a society chooses to eat must, to be sure, provide a proper nutritional balance, but they are not, as this book has shown, to be selected solely for their nutritional value. Similarly, the articles which a community decide to eat should not contain so high a concentration of toxic ingredients that the people who eat them become ill or die. At the same time, communities do not reject articles of diet which they wish to eat solely because there is some risk in eating them.

But now we come to a remarkable inconsistency in the tribal behaviour of the West. While we pay little or no attention to quite toxic foods such as cabbage and onion, rhubarb and peanuts, and smoke cigarettes and drive light-heartedly in fast cars, we make a violent clamour about what, in the jargon of technology, we describe as 'additives'. It is generally insisted that animals used to test a new additive must eat a hundred times as much of it as will ever be used in practice, and do so for their entire lifetime, that their offspring for two generations must do the same, and all be shown to have suffered no demonstrable harm, before the new stuff, whatever it may be, can be used.

[39] West, E., *Florida Agr. Exp. Sta. Circ.,* S–100, 1957.
[40] Bruce, E. A., *J. Amer. Med. Ass.,* 58, 313, 1920.

This, to say the least, is paradoxical. It is clearly necessary to take trouble to find out whether the chemical compounds we add to our foods are safe for whatever reason we add them. These reasons are in themselves diverse. Additives may be added as preservatives – that is, to prevent decay and the growth of micro-organisms; they may be used as cosmetics, to make food more beautiful and to give it colour; some are added to make loaves of bread bigger, or to make jam stiffer; to stop the oil rising to the top of mayonnaise; or the fruit pulp sinking to the bottom of the orangeade. There are additives used to give flavour and smell, or to improve the nutritional value of the article to which they are added. Some have little physiological function at all but are put in to make the legend on the label come true. The manufacturers who insist on the necessity of these things, which the harsh experience of supplying the public with what they will pay for has shown to be necessary, know what they are talking about. Food is selected for many attributes other than its nutritional value. Because additives do make foods more palatable by contributing flavour, like saccharine; rendering them more attractive in appearance, like the yellow dye added to margarine; and contributing to their nutritional value, like the chalk added to flour in Great Britain since the time of World War II, the assessment of their toxicological safety becomes important. The establishment of a rational policy by which the standard of a sensible degree of safety is to be reached is perhaps even more important. It is worth noting that an international committee of the United Nations[41] set up to think about this very problem reached the conclusion that it is impossible to establish absolute proof of the safety in use of any additive for all human beings under all conditions. Just the same, the committee reached the conclusion that properly-designed animal tests could be depended upon to assess the degree of safety – or of danger – in consuming any specified amount of one particular additive. Naturally, the committee wanted this amount to be 'substantially below any level which could be harmful to consumers'.

Proving a negative is more difficult, both technically and philo-sophically, than might be imagined. For any new chemical additive that may be proposed it is now established practice to carry out a prolonged series of tests on several different species of animals. This

[41] *First Rept.* of the Jnt. FAO/WHO Expert Committee on Food Additives, Geneva, 1966.

work involves at least two years' study, even when short-lived animals such as rats, mice or hamsters are used, and much laborious work by pathologists to examine all the tissues of the animals when they eventually die or are killed. Since there is no certainty that a substance harmful to one species of animal will affect another, even when toxic effects are found for the test animals, it does not necessarily follow that human beings would be affected, although it is prudent to assume that they would. On the other hand, it can be argued that even when substances have no effect on animals, they may still affect people. Rabbits, for example, can eat Deadly Nightshade with impunity, for they are unaffected by the atropine in it which has a powerful effect on human beings. It follows, therefore, that not even the most rigorous testing can ensure absolute safety.

Not long ago, an official American committee, the Panel on Food Additives of the President's Science Advisory Committee, reached the decision that a substance could be classified as 'safe' from potential carcinogenicity at a particular level of dosage if no cancers developed in 1,000 test animals. Three scientists, Levin, Bross and Sheehe[42] studied the mathematical basis of this test, and challenged the reliability of the committee's conclusion. They calculated that, on a statistical basis, even if a substance were in fact capable of producing 100,000 cases of cancer in a population the size of that of the United States, there would be a one in three probability that the biological test on the 1,000 animals would nevertheless classify it as 'safe'.

The pursuit of safety has been a long-drawn effort in search of what seems to be an elusive and ever-receding goal. At one time the United States authorities set out to attain the ultimate goal. They decreed that the limit for certain possibly carcinogenic compounds in food should be 'zero tolerance'. This, though a worthy ideal, was found to be a philosophical impossibility. An analyst deals with reality. He can say that the limit of sensitivity of his method is, let us say, one part per million. He cannot, if cross-questioned, say whether there may not be a lesser amount present. If his method is improved to detect whether or not one part is present in, say, ten million parts of the substance he is examining, he still can know nothing of any even smaller amount. Hence, under the terms of the US ordinance, the only way for a manufacturer to be able to market anything with a clear conscience was not to have it analysed at all.

[42] Levin, M. L., Bross, J. D., & Sheehe, P. R., *Science*, 133, 947, 1961

The history of the study of the pharmacology of food additives is full of unexpected incidents. The flour improver, Agene – the gas, nitrogen trichloride – was widely used in the United States and Great Britain for more than a generation from 1919 to 1946 to make uniform, well-risen and popular loaves. Then it was discovered by Mellanby[43] that it led to what was later found to be methionine sulphoximine being formed from the flour protein. And this substance is toxic to dogs. So Agene was dropped, and chlorine dioxide used in its place. Again, for years the oil-soluble dye, p-dimethylaminoazobenzene, so-called Butter Yellow, was included in the US list of permitted food colours. Then, in 1936, it was shown by Yoshida[44] to be capable of producing liver tumours in rats.

A different chain of events developed from the use of vitamin D, the compound, calciferol, incorporated as an additive in British welfare dried milk as a preventative against rickets. In order to ensure that each baby consumed an adequate amount, and to make allowance for any losses that might occur during processing and storage, the concentration in the National Dried Milk was gradually increased. It was then observed[45] that while the incidence of the disease, rickets, had diminished almost to vanishing-point, a new disease, so-called *ideopathic hypercalcaemia*, began to be noticed instead. The level of calciferol was thereafter reduced.

Once food scientists begin to look for danger, they find it everywhere. To ensure the harmlessness of some new additive, it may be fed to experimental animals in ever-increasing quantity until a significant proportion of their total diet is composed of the dye or emulsifier or improver of whatever may be the substance under test. If the animal finally succumbs, is the analyst to deduce that its collapse is due to the toxicity of the chemical being tested or the mortal frailty of the beast? Feeding tests to assess the possible carcinogenicity of a compound can be long-drawn-out and inconclusive. To shorten them, the tester may repeatedly inject the compound under the skin. Here again, can the investigator legitimately deduce that traces of a dye or flavouring agent eaten in a cake or sweetmeat will cause cancer, merely because an experimental animal has developed a tumour at the site of its injections? The minimum safeguard is

[43] Mellanby, E., *Brit. Med. J.*, II, 885, 1946.
[44] Yoshida, M., *Proc. Imp. Acad. Japan,* 8, 464, 1932.
[45] Lightwood, R., *Proc. Roy. Soc. Med.*, 45, 401, 1952.

117

considered to be an assessment of the incidence of tumours in two species of animals – rats and mice are a popular choice - given the compound under evaluation during their entire lifespan. An example of the difficulty of interpreting the results were the tests with the food dye, Brilliant Blue FCF, which was proved to be safe in the 'chronic oral studies' – that is, when fed – but which induced tumours when injected subcutaneously. Is it reasonable to expect food chemicals to be so safe that one can be tattooed with them with impunity?

The search for possible dangers must clearly involve the scientific study of printing inks and colours used to ornament the paper wrappings in which foods are contained. Plastic films represent one of the great advances of twentieth-century chemistry. The primary functions of wrapping foods are to preserve their 'freshness' and quality, to prevent their becoming soiled or dry, and – equally or more important – to protect them from bacterial contamination. But the plastics themselves and particularly the compounds which may be incorporated with them to improve their flexibility may migrate into the wrapped foodstuffs and present a pharmacological hazard. A considerable amount of scientific work has been done to assess the degree of contamination likely to occur, and to discover whether or not it could possibly be harmful.

In the United States, more than 2,700 different additives have been officially notified to the authorities.[46] In addition to these, however, the vast number of unintentional additives presents an even more daunting problem which constitutes the major part of the work of the US Food and Drug Administration which – at least in the opinion of some qualified observers[47] – is probably out of all proportion to the toxic hazards that such additives represent. Perhaps the most widespread kinds of unintentional additive are the modern insecticides which, to a remarkable degree, enable farmers to increase the yield of food they produce by avoiding loss and destruction by insects. These insecticides are chemical compounds which are extremely durable. Although no authenticated cases have been reported of people being poisoned because of traces of pesticides in their food, more and more of the foods eaten by the citizens of industrialized communities do, in fact, contain these substances. The chlorinated hydrocarbon pesticides, of which DDT is by far the commonest, are very persistent in

[46] Beacham, L. M., Fd. Drug Cosmetic Law J., 16, 261, 1961.
[47] Golberg, L., and Forrest, R. S., Rept. Prog. Appl. Chem., 47, 623, 1962.

soil, and are nowadays ubiquitous as residues in food crops and animal products. Recent figures for the United States[48] show that each individual in the country consumes on average 0·08 to 0·12 mg. of chlorinated organic pesticide daily. So far, the amounts swallowed are considered to be well below those likely to be harmful. For example, it is reckoned that whereas 0·5, 0·06, 9 and 1·2 micrograms of DDT, lindane, malathion and carbaryl are ingested for each kilogram of human body weight, the least amounts of these pesticides likely to be harmful are 10, 12, 14, 20 and 20 micrograms respectively.

Whether we are frightened at this situation or not, we need the extra food – and the economic advantage as well: money is excellent for relieving malnutrition – that the pesticides provide. And there is, it seems, no way on earth to be safe. It was Sladden, Menzie and Reishel[49] who first discovered that there was no place on the globe so remote from civilization that the creatures living there could escape the tide of DDT and other insecticides which, like a cloud of radioactive dust, now travels through the atmosphere and in the waters of the oceans.

Sladden, Menzie and Reishel analysed the flesh of Adelie penguins and crabeater seals captured in the Antarctic and found in their fat measurable amounts of DDT. It is interesting to note that, to obtain a 'blank' determination to verify the correctness of their analytical technique, they examined fat taken from an Emperor penguin killed over thirty years before and stored in an igloo as an emergency food supply. No DDT was detected. This could, of course, have been expected since the bird died before DDT was invented. More recently, other scientists[50] carried out a more extensive study on creatures captured on opposite sides of the Antarctic continent, in McMurdo Sound and in the Weddell Sea, and found not only DDT and its breakdown products, but BHC, heptachlor and dieldrin as well in the tissues of penguins, in penguin eggs, brown skuas – these were heavily contaminated, and blue-eyed shags; and (in the fish) notothenia.

It seems that there is no escape from danger. The conscientious food scientist in his search for nutritional excellence is confounded by

[48] Quoted by the *Food and Drugs Research Labs. Bull.*, June 1967, New York.
[49] Sladden, W. J. Z., Menzie, C. N., & Reishel, W. L., *Nature*, 210, 670, 1966.
[50] Tatton, J. O., and Ruzicka, J. H. A., *Nature*, 215, 346, 1967.

the diverse facets of human behaviour, by custom, tradition, feeling and religion, by the motives other than health which drive men to choose what they like, by the availability of foods from the land and the availability – or absence of it – of money. And now, on the other hand, in his endeavours to avoid harm from poisonous substances, the rational man is again faced with problems. The first is that he does not possess sufficient knowledge of the composition of the foods he eats, his potatoes, his peanuts and his nutmeg. The second problem is what the Americans are calling the 'benefit/risk ratio'. Among the benefits are 'the contribution of pesticides towards the production of a food supply of superior quality and sufficient quantity, the protection and preservation not only of food supplies, but of fiber, wood, textiles, the control of disease vectors, and the improvement of residential and recreational environments'. Some of the risks, I have already described.

The progress of science can be defined as the continuous minimization of doubt. The enlightened food scientist must therefore appreciate the opposing influences which he has to try to understand as he endeavours to make wise decisions.

CHAPTER IX

THE CODEX ALIMENTARIUS

The sudden invention of scientific technology little more than a century ago was without question one of the most remarkable events in the history of man. By the application of scientific knowledge to practical affairs, and by the pursuit of scientific information for specific practical objects, humanity gained a control of the natural environment of a different order of completeness from anything that had existed before. The success of the Western societies was so obvious in the field of practical affairs that their social organization and the beliefs upon which it is based spread quickly to societies which before had been organized differently. Japan, Russia, Mexico – these are among the most striking of the converts to industrialization. But as I have described in earlier chapters, other communities in Africa and Asia are absorbing the current doctrine as it spreads to its inevitable fulfilment of enveloping the whole world. In every country on earth there is a Hilton Hotel or its equivalent, and no place is so remote that a bottle of Coca-Cola cannot be found in it.

The student of food science is well aware of this. He is concerned about the intake of protein in Katmandu and the Plain of Jars in Viet Nam, just as he is with that of the people of Detroit, Marseilles and Damascus. And it is not only that in the twentieth century, with the Scientific Revolution receding into history behind us just as the French Revolution did a century or so earlier, that we are aware that all the peoples on earth have the same requirements for vitamins and proteins. These nutritional requirements must be provided in the form of foodstuffs. And in the present historical period of scientific technology, the previous diversity of foodstuffs from which different communities used to constitute their particular diets is tending to disappear and flatten out. Today, the very same articles of diet are distributed world-wide, so that an Eskimo and a bushman in the Kalahari Desert may soon both be eating powdered milk manufactured in Wisconsin, or fish fingers from a single factory in Grimsby.

The diminution in the variety of foodstuffs eaten by different communities in different parts of the world, which I have already commented upon, is merely a part of the change brought about by the spread of food technology. Another aspect of the same thing is the gradual extinction of one species of wild animal after another as the modern machine tools of agriculture subdue the ground and inexorably encroach upon every residual area of uncultivated terrain. Science applied to agriculture has, of course, been immensely successful; but its tendency has been towards uniformity, and a limitation of the variety of the animal and plant species used for food. The wheat grown on the prairies of North America is all of a specially selected genetical strain suited to the soil and climate, and resistant to the fungus diseases of smut and rust. Similarly, maize and rice, in North America, the Soviet Union, South America or Japan are only derived from seed of selected types.

But uniformity and the limitation of differences goes further than this. Scientists of the Harvard Business School have reached the conclusion that science will inevitably bring agriculture, as it has so far been understood, to an end, and cause 'agribusiness' to take its place. No longer is food produced by one set of people (farmers), sold to a second set (the wholesale dealers), packaged and marketed by a third, and very likely converted into something edible – say a pork pie or a pot of jam – by a fourth. All these operations are combined into one large-scale, streamlined, scientifically-controlled and automated manufacturing and distributing business: agribusiness. The principle was perfected by Henry Ford in 1914, and, just as there are in the whole world only a few score of different motor-cars, so there will soon be equally few kinds of staple food articles for all mankind.

Consider chickens. In 1935, about 50 million chickens were eaten in the United States; in 1965, the number was 2,300 million. Chicken meat, from being a delicacy, had become an inexpensive commonplace due directly to the application of science. Genetics had been applied to breed an appropriate strain of birds. Nutrition was employed to ensure economical growth. Pathologists ensured freedom from disease. Hens were selected and housed so as to be capable of laying 300 eggs a year. Many of the eggs were bulked and frozen to make them transportable from China to Europe or America; others were spray-dried to constitute an even more durable commodity. The handling of broilers for the table was rendered enormously more efficient by the use of mechanical and automatic devices in place of the manual processes of cottage industry. The extravagant operation

122

whereby one person killed, plucked and eviscerated a single bird, was replaced by a standardized industrial plant through which the uniform birds, killed in rapid sequence, were hung upside-down on a travelling chain by which they were transported through a series of operations in which they were plucked, washed, dissected, chilled, wrapped and finally packed for frozen transport direct to the supermarket. Inevitably, frozen chickens and standardized eggs, frozen or dried, have become industrial products manufactured for a world market by a comparatively few, big, highly capitalized and scientifically based units. And the same principle holds for sugar, tea, tobacco, bananas, margarine and other fats, cereals – the list extends, as technology moves forward to encompass the whole satellite.

It is true that there are still communities where simple, traditional diets of indigenous foods are eaten. But these communities are dwindling, and the proportions of manufactured foods (like the numbers of automobiles, bicycles, rifles and other products of technological civilization) are increasing. It was, therefore, to have been expected that, in the summer of 1963, the representatives of thirty nations, extending from Turkey to Thailand and from New Zealand to Yugoslavia, together with observers from sixteen different international organizations, should have gathered together in Rome at the headquarters of the Food and Agriculture Organization of the United Nations, to draw up a set of definitions to which the foodstuffs of scientific commerce would be compelled to conform if they were to be accepted as fit articles for international exchange. These definitions, gathered up as a Domesday Book of world eating, were to be called the Codex Alimentarius.

It is hard enough within a single country to get scientists, traders, local authorities and the general public to agree on what a fresh egg or a sausage should be. The much greater difficulty of reaching international unanimity can be seen from the fact that it took two years from the formation of the Codex Alimentarius Commission before the dates of the first meetings of some of the committees to consider different food commodities could be fixed. But whereas the first meeting on nuts – held in Ankara – was late in coming, by the time it had been held, eight sessions on milk, three on cocoa, and two each on meat, fat, sugar, and frozen foods had been arranged.

The purpose of the Codex Alimentarius Commission, to enable people the world over to know in quite precise terms the quality of the food they are buying, seems so logical that the considerable measure of progress is a significant historical event in a world of men who show all too little tendency for rational agreement. Countries which possess official standards – of food composition, of permitted colours and flavours and preservatives, or of permitted levels of trace contaminants – usually have standards that differ from each other. For example, lists of permitted food colours for one country frequently include dyes prohibited in neighbouring countries. The national standards for jam demand a minimum fruit content varying from 25 to 50 per cent. Jam, it may be argued, is not a vital article of diet; nevertheless, it demands some measure of patriotic self-restraint for those countries whose traditional jams customarily contain more or less fruit than the Codex standard to agree to meet the agreed mean minimum.

Perhaps the most remarkable feature of the very existence of the Codex is the evidence it provides of the willingness of food scientists at least to try to reach uniform conclusions after starting from different premises. There have been two attitudes. The first set out to be restrictive, to permit only what had been examined and approved. Such an attitude may be unduly conservative and hence delay innovation. Furthermore, it possesses an element of intellectual arrogance, since it implies that the licensing authority knows all that there is to know about the composition, nutritional value and freedom from toxicity of every item on the official list. The other attitude is to permit any food to be sold pending any subsequent demonstration of its harmfulness. In the United States, for example, a wide variety of foods – I hesitate to mention again potatoes, onions, rhubarb and horseradish – which would never pass the rigorous tests set up for modern innovations, are accepted as being *generally recognized as safe*. In the fashionable American language of initials, these articles are classified as GRAS.

The faith, courage and optimism of Dr Franzel, an Austrian, who in 1953 created the European Committee for Food Standards which, in 1961, was taken over by a joint committee of the Food and Agriculture Organization and the World Health Organization of the United Nations as the Codex Alimentarius, is beyond praise. Consider some of the difficulties there were – and are – to overcome.

To be of use, international agreements on the scientific nature of an item which is a traditional food in one country, must be acceptable in every other country. Yet it has been pointed out[1] that whereas, in most European countries, a sausage is a product made from minced meat, with added milk, salt and spices, in Great Britain sausages contain only 65 per cent of meat if they are called 'pork sausages', and 50 per cent if they are called 'beef sausages' – the remainder being largely wetted bread. Again, in Holland gingerbread is bread flavoured with ginger, in Great Britain, it is a sweet cake containing treacle and flavoured with ginger; while in France it is a dry, spiced and slightly sweetened cake. Then there are the Americans who call the plain cake they traditionally eat with their coffee, coffee cake. In Great Britain, however, the description, coffee cake, is reserved for a cake flavoured with coffee. Yet the British are no more logical than anyone else: a traditional article accepted as a butter puff does not contain butter, nor are cream crackers made with cream.

Staple foods in their traditional form are as difficult to define for international consumption as are some of those I have mentioned, or, for example, *chili powder* which (to an American analyst) is a mixture of a number of compounded ingredients, whereas *powdered chili* is simply chili powdered. In Great Britain and in Europe generally, powdered chili and chili powder are assumed to be the same thing. Cheese is an important and nutritious article of diet although, as we have already seen, some of its less well-known minor constitutents may exert unexpected physiological effects. Yet whereas Cheddar and Camembert cheese may be made anywhere, by anyone who knows how to make them, Cheshire cheese, to receive official approval, must be made in England, and Gorgonzola must be made in Italy.

The situation is just as complex for fish. At one time a sardine was the description of a particular fish caught off Sardinia. One problem facing the Codex Alimentarius people is, that small pilchards canned in Portugal are designated 'sardines' for part of their large international commerce. Another, that a type of sprat caught and canned by the Norwegians is also known as a sardine in America; this, in England too, is colloquially called a sardine, although the official designation is 'brisling' or 'sild'. To make matters that much more confusing, the fish that is caught off the coast of the United States and packed and marketed as a sardine in America, is actually a type of small herring.

[1] McLachlan, T., *Chem. and Ind.*, p. 174, 1963.

125

Cheese, for those who love it, is a foodstuff that has excited a curious degree of emotion, and it is interesting to note that, a decade before the Codex Alimentarius was thought of, an International Cheese Convention was signed in Stresa in Italy in 1953. The signatories were eight countries responsible for about half of the world's cheese production. The Convention prepared a list of thirty-five different kinds of cheese and laid down minimum standards of composition for each. It is interesting to note that an important provision in the Cheese Convention covered the legal enforcement by participating countries. Final authority was vested in the International Court of Justice in The Hague. It is a happy thought that whether or no this august body can effectively arbitrate a peaceful passage through the Straits of Tiran, or the rights of the Buganda of Burundi, at least its ruling on the amount of fat in Roquefort cheese carries the weight of law.

The fact that an International Cheese Convention could be set up and could to a large degree actually function, led to the holding of a Conference on Food Standards under the joint auspices of the Food and Agriculture Organization and the World Health Organization in Geneva in October, 1962. In spite of the diverse unsettled problems between the nations of the world, this conference courageously recommended the establishment of the Codex Alimentarius Commission, outlined its rules, and enjoyed the satisfaction of seeing its first session held in Rome in June and July, 1963. The Commission elected for itself an American chairman and three vice-chairmen (one from the Netherlands, one from New Zealand and one from Poland), and called six nations to provide representatives to serve on its executive committee. These were Argentina, Australia, Canada, India, Senegal and the United Kingdom. Here, then, we had an international gathering with members drawn from Europe, Asia, North America, South America, Africa and Australasia – every inhabited continent of the world – whose purpose was to specify in scientific terms foodstuffs from major articles like flour, to minor items such as soup cubes, so that all peoples could benefit from their nutriments.

The organization of the Codex Alimentarius was set up in a highly professional way. First, broad standards would be established so that a lowest common denominator, as it were, for, say, cheese or groundnut-oil would be recognized. Later, work would be done to specify

126

what was meant by 'full fat cheese', 'skimmed milk cheese' and 'refined groundnut oil'. Later still, details were laid down of what could
legitimately be added to cheese and groundnut-oil without overstep-
ping the definition of each; and how these and other items should be
labelled for possible distribution throughout the world.[2]

The first duties of the Codex Alimentarius Commission were to
study what had been done before to set up standards for the world's
food. There was work already completed by an Expert Commission
on Food Additives which had reported to the United Nations. There
were the labours of an earlier European Codex Alimentarius Council
to consider. A committee of experts was chosen to take account of
what had been done by an FAO Working Party and a WHO Expert
Committee – the difference between a working party and an expert
committee is a subtle one – on Pesticide Residues. Then, having
taken steps to get the measure of what other people had done, the
commissioners of the Codex Alimentarius planned their own work.
They set up one Expert Committee under the chairmanship of a
Dutchman to consider food additives, another under a Canadian to
think about pesticide residues, and a third with a Canadian at the
head to decide what to do about labels. More experts were collected
to study methods for analysing foods, and for setting up standards of
hygiene for everything except meat, milk and products derived from
milk – these being left to the United Nations' committees to deal
with. The British were set to be chairman of the Expert Committee
for fats and oils, although margarine was left to the International
Federation of Margarine Associations, and olive oil to the International Olive Council.

Of the other main foodstuffs, meat was to be studied by an Expert
Committee with Federal Germany in the chair; poultry was left to the
Americans to discuss; standards for fresh and canned fish were made
the business of the British; and those for wheat were left to the
International Organization for Standardization. A Working Party of
the E.C.E. (Economic Commission for Europe) had just completed
work on standards for market fruit; but for processed fruit and
vegetables, and such things as tomato purée, jam, currants, raisins
and prunes, a special Expert Committee was set up with the United
States in the chair. Even such apparently insignificant food items as
fruit juices of diverse sorts were taken account of by the Codex

[2] Blanchfield, J. R., *Food Manufacture*, 40, 39, 1965.

Alimentarius Commission. Draft standards for apple-juice, orange-juice and grape-juice set up by an Expert Group – not an Expert Committee this time – working in collaboration with the European Economic Committee, were circulated so that other nations could comment on them; while another Expert Group consulted with the European Codex Alimentarius Council and with the authors of the Latin-American Food Code and a group of experts from the European Economic Committee, to formulate standards for – of all things – edible fungi.

What more was there to do for a start? There were draft coding standards for cocoa beans, prepared by a Study Group of the Food and Agriculture Organization, to consider; and an Expert Committee on Cocoa Products and Chocolate to set up under the chairmanship of a Swiss. The British looked after an Expert Committee on sugar and all kinds of sweetening matter except honey. This was reserved for another Expert Committee under the chairmanship of an Austrian. Finally, Czechoslovakia, having proposed that world standards for soft drinks and beer should be worked out, the Commission decided to defer any consideration about beer; and then, after having pondered the views of Great Britain on soft drinks, decided to defer any decision on these as well. Eggs too were deferred as being too difficult to standardize.

Yet the amount of effort deployed to launch this major project in science-based human endeavour was indeed formidable. Consider that statement of general principles drawn up for the governments of the European nations taking part. This began characteristically with comments about what an analyst should do if he thought an article was not properly labelled – that is, that the expectations held out by the label were not fulfilled when the consumer unwrapped the package. There were sections describing what was to be understood by a foodstuff injurious to health. Included in this part of the statement was a passage pointing out that, if a consumer injured his health by 'excessive or unreasonable consumption of a foodstuff' – for example, by gross and continuous over-eating or (and this was explicitly stated and is, indeed, a well-known method of damaging one's health) intemperate and excessive consumption of intoxicating beverages – it must be taken as his own fault: the quality of the food and drink could not be held to blame. Then again, some people are specially sensitive to particular foods. There are those who come out

128

in a rash when they eat strawberries or oysters. Under these circumstances of so-called allergy, the quality of the food obviously cannot be held responsible. On the other hand, there may be cases when an item in the form in which it is prepared as an article of international commerce would in fact be harmful. For example, preserved fruit containing comparatively high concentrations of sulphur dioxide is a common item of trade. In this instance, it is considered proper to approve of its trans-shipment, but, at the same time, to make it the business of the supplier to warn the consumer not to eat it until the excess sulphur dioxide has been driven off. This takes place, for example, during the process by which such fruit is converted into jam.

The working out of precise specifications for the great variety of food items which appear in world commerce is clearly a laborious, difficult and slow business. Even for any *one* country to determine what the acceptable limits of composition should be, is a difficult enough problem in both science and economics. High quality – even if it can be defined – is a desirable target, but to forbid what might be considered inferior standards could readily be to the disadvantage of poorer communities for whom half a loaf would be better than no bread. The problem when many nations with different tastes and customs and different economic standards are involved, is infinitely more puzzling. It is little wonder that much of the work of the Codex Alimentarius Commission was consumed in procedural matters and statements of generalities.

Significant sections of the statement of principles with which the group of European nations found themselves wrestling[3] concern the recognition of micro-organisms capable of causing food poisoning, of adulterants, and of toxic substances. There was a further section in which spoilage was defined – no easy matter when, for example, meat considered to be decayed and uneatable by one group of people in one part of the world might be accepted as attractively 'high' in another. As the text points out, even spoiled food can be edible. Nevertheless, an article can be taken as officially spoiled if it has reached a condition 'so far from the consumer's justified expectations that it has partly or wholly lost its usefulness' or if it has been 'processed in a way which would arouse the disgust of the average

[3] Joint FAO/WHO Codex Alimentarius Commission, *Rept*, of the First Session, Rome, 1963.

consumer . . . if he were aware of these circumstances'. No one reading this draft can fail to admire the evangelical enthusiasm of the members of the Codex Commission in their task of establishing parity of disgust throughout the world.

A second draft code drawn up by the Latin-American nations came to much the same conclusions, but by a different route. First, the more logical Latin-American experts defined consumers. They are people who procure food for personal consumption, or for consumption by a third party. Then food was redefined. It is not only a substance which when ingested supplies the body with something for its biological processes, but it is also to include those materials added to foods the consumption of which is 'customary or pleasurable'. Clearly, this must include on both counts the silver thimbles incorporated in Christmas puddings.

The definition went on to say that in this sense solid, liquid and gaseous substances can all be food. Should the reference to gaseous materials eventually be ratified, it will be perhaps the first time that an official, scientifically-based definition of food has been extended to include such essential components of quality as the aroma of frying bacon and the bubbles in champagne.

Yet it is not altogether surprising after all. Scientific assessment of food includes more than its chemical composition. We have already seen that it comprises its smell, which comes within the ambit of the clause covering 'parity of disgust'. The firmness or toughness of foodstuffs is also a relevant measure of their quality; rheology is the branch of science which has been developed to measure and describe such characteristics. The appearance, and particularly the colour, of foods are topics upon which much research has been done, and serious consideration has been paid to the assessment of possible danger from the use of dyes. Colour has little or no bearing on the nutritional value of food; yet people are prepared to submit to by no means negligible risk for the aesthetic, evanescent view of green canned peas, yellow margarine and multi-coloured ice-cream. It is reasonable, therefore, that in spite of the differences between the lists of dyes accepted as safe by different member countries, the Codex Alimentarius Commission should do their best to draw up an agreed selection.

Composition, appearance as judged by eye, consistency measured by touch, flavour by taste, and aroma by smell – all these are characteristics which can be assessed scientifically. Even hearing plays a part in food quality. Celery, potato crisps and toast must, it seems, produce the appropriate noise. In 1963 a Swedish scientist, Birger Drake, carried out a study at the Quartermaster Food and Container Institute for the Armed Forces in the United States to measure 'food crunching sounds'.[4] The amplitude, frequency and duration of the sounds produced by masticating such items as crisp brown bread, lettuce, ham, apples, tough beef and peanuts were recorded on magnetic tape and precisely measured. In a later research,[5] the technique was further refined and the study continued. The final conclusions provide a good example of the way in which the widening scope of food technology is advanced:

> Taken together, the results indicate that an extended study of mastication sounds could be of value in food technology, especially after further improvements of the technique. Such work should be focused on qualitative differences, which could be expected to supplement the present results of a more quantitative nature. Such differences would probably be more closely related to frequencies and/or durations of sounds than to their amplitudes.

This is merely one example of the multiplicity of topics into which food technologists penetrate. So far, noise has not entered into the international discussion of food composition. Just the same, the diversity of detail with which the Codex Commission are attempting to deal is very great. To start from a statement of general principle seems simple. Yet even the four principles drawn up as justification for the use of food additives can be seen to present subtle problems. The first, that additives should improve nutritional quality, is unexceptionable. The next, that they should 'enhance the keeping quality or stability with resulting reduction in food wastage' may be well enough. Yet the history of food science contains incidents in which preservatives have not invariably been welcome additions to food. It falls, therefore, to the wise men of the Codex Alimentarius to amplify their principle by lists of approved preservatives and statutory limits in their use. The third principle offers even more knotty doctrinal problems. It states that food additives can be justified provided they make 'foods attractive to the consumer in a manner which does not

---

[4] Drake, B. K., *J. Food Sci.*, 28, 233, 1963.
[5] Drake, B. K., *J. Food Sci.*, 30, 556, 1965.

lead to deception'. Does the addition of yellow dye to a cake lead the consumer to believe that it contains egg? And should a really convincing raspberry flavour be developed, will its use be wrong in the absence of raspberries?

The fourth principle to govern the use of additives is most difficult of all. They can be approved if they are 'essential aids in food processing'. It is no wonder that the text of the Commission's drafts is long, as are also the lists of 'antimicrobial preservatives', 'antioxidants and synergists', and 'emulsifiers and stabilizers'.

The Codex Alimentarius commissioners have set out to apply their scientific criteria in considerable detail to the world's articles of food. Let us, as an example, consider their standards for apples and pears. These standard apply 'to dessert and culinary apples and pears, being fresh fruit grown from varieties of *Pyrus Malus L.* and *Pyrus Communis L.*'. To start with, the fruit must be 'intact', 'sound', 'clean', 'free from all abnormal external moisture' and 'free from foreign smell and taste'. Next, 'the fruit must be carefully hand-picked and sufficiently developed'. Then comes a description of various grades. For example, 'Extra Class: fruit in this class must be of superlative quality.' Then there are 'Class I' and 'Class II' and so on. To tomatoes, *Lycoperisicum Esculentum Mill*, cauliflowers, *Brassica Oleracea L., Variety botrytis L.,* onions, lettuces, curled-leaved endives and broad-leaved (Batavian) endives, peaches, apricots and plums, and, indeed to a long list of foods, the same kind of thing applies. For each there are grades and sub-grades, specified sizes and colours, instructions about packing, regulations about labelling. For grapes, there are long lists of varieties grown in open ground, some large-berry varieties, some small-berry varieties, and other lists of hothouse varieties. Lemons 'other than verdelli' must contain a minimum juice content of 25 per cent. Verdelli lemons – primo fiore – need only contain 20 per cent of juice to reach the minimum specification.

Meticulously the Codex commissioners particularize the colour, shape and juice content of clementines, mandarines, satsumas, wilkings, oranges, grapefruit or pomelos. They review the composition of mineral waters and dietetic foods, and discuss the reports of the International Federation of Soup Manufacturers on the desirable composition of broths and soups.[6] Divergent views about edible ices

[6] Codex Alimentarius Commission, *Rept*, of the Fourth Session, Rome, 1966.

and ice-cream were reviewed by a Co-ordinating Committee directed by the Swedish delegation; while the comments of a number of European and non-European governments on the definition of 'dirty honey', the analysis of water-insoluble solids in honey, the acidity of honey, and the significance of diastase and hydroxymethyl furfural (HMF) in honey, were submitted to another Coordinating Committee appointed for the purpose.

Applied science has made the world small, to be sure, and many people in the world eat food grown and processed with the help of technological processes based on science. Without these science-based processes they would eat less well or not at all. Yet, as it has been the purpose of this book to show, science has its limits. Much is to be hoped from the devoted work of the Codex Alimentarius Commission setting up rational standards for quality, chemical composition, permitted additives and limits for bacterial contamination for the world's food commodities. Much is to be expected from all this, but not too much.

As I see it, there are two limits to the possibilities inherent in the ideas underlying the Codex Alimentarius. The first arises from considerations of human psychology, that is, the nature of man; and, in particular, the nature of the food scientists and administrators who are working out the various world standards. The second limit is the incompleteness of scientific knowledge.

It is customary to assume that a scientist is possessed of an ice-cold intelligence, unbiased by emotion, and influenced only by scientific evidence. This is not true in two respects. Firstly, two equally competent scientists may interpret the same set of facts in almost exactly opposite ways. I have already pointed out that one scientist may logically deduce that a man consuming 16 mg. of ascorbic acid (vitamin C) daily is obtaining enough to satisfy his physiological demands; another may classify such an individual as malnourished. We have also seen that tests which purport to show that 100 times the normal level of consumption of a particular additive are a certain assurance of its safety in use, may not, in fact, ensure that this is so. Furthermore, scientists who insist on testing new foods at the level of 100 times the normal intake, see no illogic in accepting very much more common foods which they know to be toxic at levels of only three or four times the customary levels of consumption.

A more fundamental fallibility of food scientists – and one to

133

which reference is never made in respectable circles – is that they share with all the rest of humanity the temptation to be dishonest. I am not suggesting that there are many scientists who put forward experimental results they know to be false. It is, nevertheless, a wise legal precaution not to allow a man to be a judge in his own cause. It is equally prudent to consider rather carefully the conclusions of a scientist – or a group of like-minded scientists – who are known to have held particular views on a matter *before* they carried out the scientific studies which were designed to demonstrate that those views were correct. No one doubts the moral integrity of the American public-health authorities who set up the so-called 'filth test' which condemned the import of biscuits from abroad if mouse-hairs were detected in them, no matter how few. The fact that the imported biscuits could have been troublesome competitors for United States manufacturers was only an incidental consideration. A similar example was the prohibition for many years of colouring matter in US margarine. It could be argued that artificial colouring matter might be a toxic hazard, and, furthermore, could deceive the consumer. It is now admitted that the primary purpose of the regulation was to protect the powerful American dairying industry by compelling the margarine-makers to market their product as an unattractive white fat.

F. D. Ommanney[7] in discussing the application of Western scientific methods to sea-fishing in tropical areas, drew attention to the fact that local governments in south-east Asia and elsewhere do not always seem to believe in the integrity of the scientists they employ. In this instance, it is not necessarily that the scientists are dishonest. The distrust is due rather to a difference in aim. For whereas the local authority is paying money for the services of a scientific consultant from whom they expect to get something back which can be evaluated in terms of cash within a reasonable period of time, the scientific workers are interested in conducting research, the results of which they cannot foresee, and which in the end may not produce any result at all of monetary significance. As Ommanney put it: 'Unfortunately to guarantee a useful return is not possible with scientific research, the results of which are often unforeseeable and intangible.'

No one doubts that the scientists and food technologists who are

[7] Ommanney, F. D., *The Better Use of the World's Fauna for Food*, Inst. Biol. London, p. 95, 1963.

working so hard for the Codex Alimentarius to establish standards of food quality acceptable the world over are spurred on by the highest motives. Nevertheless, part of their purpose is to encourage trade, and trade not only in wheat and rice, canned meat and other staple articles for want of which men may starve, but also in honey and edible fungi and extra-special grades of tomatoes by which traders may become rich. The values by which technological nations live are extending widely across the world, and the reaction of Western orientated peoples to the stimulus of breakfast-foods and canned salmon have as much ethnological significance as have the articles of tribal diets in less sophisticated parts of the earth on the behaviour of the people who live there. It is, therefore, important for the food scientist to take note of the report of the Fourth Session of the Codex Alimentarius Commission held in Rome in November 1966. Here it was stated that when six African countries were asked whether they favoured the setting-up of a Co-ordinating Committee for Africa, five did not answer and the sixth withdrew. As the body committed to spreading the idea of the Codex Alimentarius to all mankind, the Commission, while agreeing in the light of this response that 'it would be premature to take any decision to propose the setting up of a Co-ordinating Committee for Africa,' did recommend FAO on every occasion to preach the value of the Codex at 'regional meetings and seminars' in Africa.

But even if it becomes possible to guarantee that the motives of the people who set the standards are pure, there still remains the fact that scientific knowledge will always be incomplete. And because this is so, the notion of a world-wide standard needs thoughtful scrutiny.

Golberg[8] has drawn attention to the implications of so simple a food ingredient as caramel. Public health authorities and pharmacologists have given much scrutiny to the possibility that so-called diazo (coal-tar dyes) could cause cancers. For this reason, those substances included in official lists of permitted food colours have been submitted to exhaustive animal tests. Caramel, however, was always accepted without hesitation as a safe colouring matter. Traditionally, caramel was produced by heating sugar or starch. Its manufacture was basically a cooking process similar in principle to roasting coffee or peanuts. But with the introduction of large-scale industrial manufacture, caramel for distribution all over the world was made with the

[8] Golberg, L., *J. Roy. Coll. Physicians*, London, I, 385, 1967.

FOOD AND SOCIETY

use of acids, alkalis or various salts. The United States authorities recognize some twenty alternative processes. The British Standard No. 3874 of 1965 covers the 'action of heat . . . in the presence or absence of acids or alkalis or of combinations of these'. A widely-used form of caramel is made by heating glucose and ammonia under pressure. Three Japanese scientists, Fujii, Tsuchida and Komoto,[9] identified five imidazole derivatives in caramel of this type, while glucosylamine, di-glucosylamine and other heterocyclic products including pyrazines may also be present. The point is that caramel, manufactured on an industrial scale (as foods must increasingly be in the technological world of the twentieth century), distributed widely, and of a composition approved by international authority nevertheless contains components the physiological effect of which is unknown.

In the main, the existence of an informed altruistic international body – the Codex Alimentarius Commission – will do good and is to be welcomed by food scientists. The dwindling size of the globe, which can now be circumnavigated in ninety minutes, and the increasing scale of the operations of a single food-manufacturer, make it important that minimum standards at least be established. At the same time, science knows no end. The knowledge of one day is only the minimization of doubt for the next. There will be more knowledge to come. The international regulations will, therefore, be dangerous if they are too restrictive; perhaps there is a danger, too, if they gain currency without challenge over the whole world.

Cabbage contains a harmful goitre-producing component; further research showed that rutabaga, turnip, peach, pear, strawberry, spinach and carrot do as well.[10] Peanuts contaminated by mould may contain a cancer-producing toxin; so may rice,[11] cycad nuts[12] and safrole[13] – which for many years, as oil of sassafras, was used in quasi-medicinal drinks. Nutmeg contains hallucinogenic compounds with pronounced toxic properties;[14] so does Jimson weed which is

[9] Fujii, S., Tsuchida, H., and Komoto, M., *Agr. Biol. Chem.*, 30, 73, 1966.
[10] Greer, M. A., *Physiol. Rev.*, 30, 513, 1950.
[11] Kobayashi, G., *et. al.*, *Proc. Japan Acad.*, 35, 501, 1959.
[12] Laqeur, G. L., Michelsen, O., Whiting, M. G., & Kurland, L. T., *J. Nat. Cancer Inst.*, 31, 919, 1963.
[13] Hamburger, F., Kelley, T., Baker, T. R., & Russfield, A. B., *Arch. Pathol.*, 73, 118, 1962.
[14] Weiss, G. *Psychiat. Quart.*, 34, 346, 1960.

frequently consumed, and does harm, in the United States.[15] Several outbreaks of honey-poisoning have occurred in New Zealand; this has been traced to the bees having collected nectar from the tutu plant, *Coriaria arborea*.[16]

The list could be extended much further. Nature is full of surprises. No scientist can know everything. But the New Zealand honey which poisoned a few people in New Zealand could, when the Codex Alimentarius is accepted as giving the certificate of approval for the distribution of a standard article from a single supplier throughout the whole world, poison many more. And if honey, why not milk also? Tremetol is an unusual compound, an unsaturated alcohol, which is known to occur in only two plants, *Eupatorium urticaepholium* and *Apolopapus heterophyllus*, white snakeroot. It is believed[17] that Abraham Lincoln's mother died when he was seven years old from drinking milk from a cow that had eaten white snakeroot.

[15] Jacobzina, H., & Reybin, H. W., *N.Y. State J. Med.,* 60, 3139, 1960.

[16] Melville, A., & Fastiev, F. N., *Proc. U. Otago Med. School,* 42, 3, 1964.

[17] Hartmann, A. F., Purkerson, M. L., & Wesley, M. E., *J. Amer. Med. Ass.,* 185, 706, 1963.

CHAPTER X

HEALTH AND NUTRITIONAL SCIENCE

The relation of nutritional knowledge to health can be considered at a number of levels. First, scientific knowledge can be applied to one particular person. The physiological requirements of an individual at any particular point of time can be established with considerable precision. His calorie needs can be assessed directly by measuring his energy expenditure, and this is commonly done in scientific studies. The patient must, however, be 'piped up' for the purpose, hung round with the necessary instruments, and observed for every moment of the day and night. An indirect method for measuring calorie requirements is to determine the calorific content of the food and drink consumed, and to make a careful and continuous watch of body-weight. If the weight remains constant, the amount of calories ingested is sufficient to cover the amount of energy expended. The adequacy or otherwise of the protein in an individual's diet can be judged by similar scientific means. This time, the measurements must include an analysis of the amount of protein consumed, and a parallel assessment of the nitrogen determined from protein-breakdown excreted in urine. More precise study must extend to investigation not merely of the protein, but of the constituent amino acids of which it is composed.[1] After two generations of studies of this sort, information has been collected about the needs of different people and different types of people – men and women, children of various ages, pregnant women, athletes – not only for calories and protein, but for an extended list of vitamins and mineral nutrients as well. Individuals vary a good deal from each other, a few are born with quite striking biochemical anomalies. People of different physical types – ectomorphs, endomorphs and mesomorphs[2] – also tend to differ in their nutritional requirements. Nevertheless, it is a comparatively straightforward, albeit laborious, task to determine the optimum diet in terms of nutrients for any particular individual should there be a sufficiently strong motive to make the effort worth while – if, for example, the

[1] FAO. Nutritional Studies, No. 16, Rome, 1957.
[2] Sheldon, W. H., *The Varieties of human physique*, Harper, New York, 1940.

man were an astronaut preparing to set out for a fortnight in a cabin the size of a telephone box.

A different level of inquiry is needed to assess the nutritional requirements for health of a group or community of people. We are now dealing, not with a special individual, but with an average man or woman. Again, a considerable body of scientific knowledge is available. During the thirty-odd years from the 1930s to the 1960s, estimates were drawn up by people best qualified to judge of recommended amounts of calories and of a continually extending list of nutrients, the consumption of which by the members of a specified group would, it was alleged, maintain them in full nutritional health. The proposed lists date from that of the League of Nations in 1935,[3] of Steibling in 1953,[4] of successive Committees of the US National Research Council,[5] of the British Medical Association,[6] of the Indian Nutrition Advisory Committee,[7] and of many others, up to those of the Food and Agriculture Organization of the United Nations.[8]

Although these schedules of nutritional intake serve a useful purpose, their value is limited in three directions. Firstly, since they are mostly recommendations of amounts known to be in excess of the levels at which recognizable deficiency could ever be expected to occur, they are often wastefully generous. And by overestimating real needs they may come to mislead worthy people – private citizens possessed of social conscience and administrators alike – who readily come to equate the number of individuals whose diet falls short of the official tables by no matter how little, with the number of people in the community suffering from 'hunger'. It is always damaging to cry wolf too often.

The second limitation of lists of recommended nutritional allowances applied to a mixed community of people is, that even when the total amount of food provides the *average* amounts of calories, vitamins, minerals and protein recommended, there is no insurance that the distribution of food within the community provides each

[3] League of Nations Tech. Commission, *Rept. of the physiological bases of nutritions*, A, 12(a), IIB, 1936.
[4] Steibling, H. K., US Dept. Agric, Misc. Pub., 183, 1953.
[5] US National Res. Council, Food and Nutrition Board, Rept. and Circular Ser., 115, 1943; 122, 1945; 129, 1948; 589, 1958.
[6] *Rept. of the Committee on Nutrition*, 1950.
[7] Indian Nutr. Advisory Committee, *Report*, 1944.
[8] FAO Nutritional Studies, 5, 1950; 19, 1957; 16, 1957.

member with his needs. Not enough crumbs may always fall from the rich man's table to supply the needs of the beggar at his gate, even if the beggar is allowed to come and eat them. For large and complex social communities such, for example, as the population of India, recommended nutrient allowances, though useful, may give a seriously inadequate picture which may be too favourable for one Indian or too unfavourable for another. Apart from different classes in a community, the problem of ensuring that vulnerable individuals within a family group receive adequate nutrition for health, is well recognized. Many of the children suffering from the protein deficiency, kwashiorkor, are victims of the social arrangements necessitating their being weaned from their mothers on the conception of a new baby.

The third shortcoming of relating the total nutrient-content of the food supplies available to a community, with their average requirements, arises from the fact that people eat foods, they do not ingest nutrients. And, as we have already seen from the earlier chapters of this book, people may not always choose to eat the foods offered to them no matter how nourishing they may be.

Nutritional science can be applied with some confidence of success to ensure the health of special categories of individuals such as athletes, soldiers, criminals in jail or indentured workers in gold mines. Such groups are substantially homogeneous, and usually include human beings at a certain fixed period in their development. The feeding of athletes to ensure nutritional health is in many respects as easy as the provision of nutritionally adequate rations for pigs and cattle that are required to be in prime condition at one particular date. Its relative simplicity is not only due to the homogeneity of the group, but also to the absence of that complexity and variety of biological behaviour that makes up a complete living human society.

The main inadequacy of much of the current corpus of knowledge that makes up the science of nutrition is that it applies only to a particular period of time. Just as it is important to use knowledge of the chemical composition of food, and the physiological function of the chemical substances of which food is composed, in the context of human behaviour as a whole, so also is it necessary to relate the knowledge of nutrition to an individual in the dimensions of his lifetime. At one time it was accepted nutritional doctrine that, if an individual failed to obtain a diet reckoned to be adequate by reference to one or other of the tables of official recommendations – for no matter how short a time – he would suffer from a permanent nutritional scar. This view is no longer tenable. For example, Ellis[9] made a study of Belgian messenger-boys whose growth was severely restricted by malnutrition during the years of World War II, but who quickly caught up with their contemporaries when adequate food became available. On the other hand, the smaller stature of working-class Glasgow children compared with the better physique of pupils in the English schools for upper middle-class boys, implies that an unsatisfactory diet continued for too long a time will, as might be expected, exert a permanent effect on physique, if not on health.

The most remarkable evidence that nutrition may exert an effect on the span of life was discovered by Clive McCay and his colleagues,[10] not for men but for rats. These workers showed that if too generous a diet was given to young rats, so that their growth and maturity were accelerated, their life span was shortened. Although many of the people concerned with human nutrition, who like to see children growing faster than their parents grew, and who take pride in watching the effect of pints of milk and plates of meat on the size and physique of boys and girls as if they were prize livestock, have denied the relevance of McCay's findings on rats to the physiology of children, it may indeed apply. For example, McCance[11] has pointed out that the physiological age of the bones of children who have been given an ample diet with supplementary milk to encourage their growth, is significantly older than that of children who have grown less quickly. The age of one's bones is a significant pointer to physiological age, and the death of old people is frequently heralded by the breaking of one of their bones. Besides the evidence obtained by radiography, the acceleration of maturity by high levels of feeding early in life which is so characteristically seen in the children of the well-fed West, can also be cited as a further possible indication that 'super' nutrition may in fact shorten life.

In considering the question of nutrition, health and the span of life, modern scientists usually neglect the phenomenon of senescence. The

[9] Ellis, R. W. B., *Arch. Dis. Childh.*, 21, 181, 1946.
[10] McCay, C. M., Maynard, L. A., Sperling, G., and Barnes, L. Z., *J. Nutrition*, 18, 1, 1939.
[11] McCance, R. A., *Lancet* II, 739, 1953.

real difficulty in discussing the problem of nutrition and health at all in its modern context, is that the definition of health accepted by the modern technological world, as represented by the World Health Organization,[12] as 'a state of complete physical, mental and social wellbeing and not merely the absence of disease or infirmity', is unattainable in this vale of tears even with the help of technology. Gordon,[13] for one, has cogently argued that the idea of 'complete physical, mental and social wellbeing' is unrealistic. A man is an organism which is continuously evolving and which is at all times in a precariously-balanced state of dynamic equilibrium with his environment. To maintain his equilibrium, as we have already seen, man and his species are in perpetual struggle – with microbes, with his family, his workmates, his employer and with the climate. Biochemically, his cells maintain an equilibrium with the nutrients of his diet. The reduction in basal metabolic rate that occurs when the energy-value of the diet falls, is a well-known adjustment; and it is difficult to decide whether, as the conventional dietician would assert, this state of equilibrium ought always to be considered 'malnutrition'. Similarly, a foetus nourished from a maternal bloodstream containing less vitamin A than, let us say, that derived from a diet recommended by the US National Research Council, might successfully adjust itself to its environment, and develop into a man of genius rather than just one more 65-kilogram 'reference man'.

The main reason why 'health' as officially defined is an unattainable goal, is because the state of equilibrium in which a man maintains himself in his environment must be constantly adjusted as time passes. The body dies a little every day, and no diet, be it ever so nutritious, can stop it. Shock[14] has pointed out that the performance of the lungs, heart and kidneys deteriorates, certainly from the age of thirty and probably before. The elasticity of the skin is obviously less from one decade to the next. Brain cells die and are not replaced, so that the average weight of the brain diminishes by 11 per cent between the ages of thirty and ninety. The average number of taste buds in each papilla of the tongue falls from 245 to 88 during these same sixty years of a man's life. Hence, if the cake a mother baked for her son could in fact be preserved without change until he was an old man,

[12] WHO International Health Conference, New York, 1946.
[13] Gordon, J., *Lancet*, II, 638, 1958.
[14] Shock, N. W., *Sci. American*, 206, 100, 1962.

he would still assert that it was not as good as what 'mother used to bake'.

These changes in the different types of cells in the body present a problem to the nutritionist. To what extent are the decalcification of the bones, the loss of elasticity of the skin, the reduction in the efficiency of the muscles, the kidneys and the lungs, and the death of the cells of the tongue and the brain, departures from health? Are these any concern of the food scientist and the nutritional expert?

Discoveries in nutrition made largely during the present twentieth century have contributed substantial benefits to humanity. In 1916, the cause and treatment of rickets were unknown. As a boy, I watched a nurse rubbing my younger sister's legs with olive oil to prevent rickets and ensure that the bones should grow straight. It was only in 1926 that Corry Mann[15] published the results of the study in which he had shown that the health and physique of boys in an orphanage, which was notably well run according to the nutritional knowledge of the times, were demonstrably improved when the children were given a daily glass of milk rather than some other supplement to their normal diet.

Within little more than a generation, scientific knowledge of nutrition has given those who possess it great power. It is not my purpose to denigrate the value of this knowledge. Distinguished men and women have made great dicoveries. Hopkins, Peters, Chick, Mellanby and Drummond in Great Britain; Steenbock, McCallum, Goldberger, Elvehjem and King in the United States; Jansen in Holland; Szent-Gyorgyi in Hungary – the list could be extended much longer. The power of the scientific discoveries of nutrition is great, but much of it deals only with the limited area of the chemical composition of food, and the biochemical mechanisms by which the human body functions. Many of the other factors which bear on the behaviour of men and of the higher animals, of which man constitutes so very special a case, are outside nutrition.

Nutrition comprises a substantial corpus of knowledge which can be taught didactically. Nevertheless, because the very nature of science is that the hypotheses constructed by each generation of workers must always be doubted by subsequent generations and consequently be subjected to test in the light of new knowledge as it

[15] Corry Mann, H. C., Med. Res. Council, *Sp. Rep. Ser.*, 104, 1926.

143

accrues, to teach a scientific subject to people who do not understand what science is about presents very peculiar difficulties.

These difficulties are in certain respects even more formidable in technologically advanced communities than they are in those less familiar with Western attitudes of thinking. In a society where beri-beri is rife and where people can be seen to suffer and die from it, the lesson that parboiled rice is better for health than polished rice can be learned comparatively easily. But in wealthier and more sophisticated countries where beri-beri is never seen, teaching about the relative concentrations of thiamine (vitamin B_1) in brown bread and white bread, polyneuritis in rats, co-carboxylase in muscle tissues, and the accumulation of pyruvic acid in blood – all germane to the mechanism of vitamin B_1-deficiency – are calculated rather to enhance the moral satisfaction of the teacher than contribute to the health of the community.

Good teachers are aware that their business has two parts: the first is to convey information, but the second is to give understanding and thereafter to influence the learner to take appropriate action. In teaching nutrition, information is essential to understanding. At the same time, there are those who acquire information without under-standing. And the commonest cause of failure to understand is to lack comprehension of what constitutes science. Consider the convert to nutrition who has been taught that salad is rich in vitamin C and that cooking destroys it, and who, in consequence, preaches to hungry coalminers who never had a day's scurvy in their lives that their health would be improved if they ate lettuce rather than steak-and-kidney-pudding, potatoes and boiled cabbage. And who has not heard a too-well-taught pupil who has learned without comprehen-sion, recommending others to eat carrots if they wish to see in the dark, take vitamin C to cure a cold, drink more milk if the Govern-ment posters say so, and go to work on an egg?

Up till the present time, much nutritional teaching has been done didactically. Children at school have been expected to accept what the teacher teaches and what the books say. Students in colleges of 'domestic science' have usually been asked to do the same. In recent years there has, however, been a change in approach to the teaching of biology – of which nutrition is, of course, a part. The new emphasis is on observation and experiment rather than on the memorizing of facts. By stressing the dependence of biological knowledge on observation and trial, the teacher can show by inference that biology is a science; in doing this, the good teacher can also teach that nutrition is only a minor province of biology, which itself covers the whole diverse and complex scene of animate creation.

Didactic, authoritarian instruction has a place where there is an immediate job to be done and where the people taught can see that this is so, have confidence in the wisdom and honesty of their teacher, and are eager to learn. A serious-minded expectant mother will benefit from instruction about calcium and vitamin D. Later, when her baby is born, she will continue to listen to instruction about 'body-building' and 'protective' foods. The inexperienced but earnest mother is actively seeking for nutritional knowledge for her baby which she can see growing or ceasing to grow week by week. But once the pressure is removed, the 'oh-so-easy-to-take', 'instant' knowledge of didactic nutrition teaching loses its virtue. And its virtue may be lost both for the teacher and the taught.

During World War I, the British public were exposed to a considerable pressure of 'education' on the subject of food. There is still to be seen in the Imperial War Museum a typical picture of a housewife standing in front of a coal-fired kitchen range and gazing through the legend: 'The kitchen is the key to victory, EAT LESS BREAD.' Not a very high level of nutritional science, it can be said, even for 1917. Another exhortation of a somewhat more intellectual level was designed to persuade the public to follow what were later seen to be the ill-advised calculations of Sir Thomas Chisholm, – a big-wig of the time – whose daily ration – so ran the poster – consisted of a plate of porridge and two slices of bread for breakfast; macaroni and cheese for lunch; a slice of bread for tea; and soup, 3 ounces of meat, half a slice of bread, and rice-pudding for dinner – plus tea or coffee without milk or sugar. Even in the distant days of 1917 and 1918, however, there was a poster of 'twenty-four common foods comparing the nourishment contained in 1 lb. weight of each' in terms of moisture, calories, and protein.

When the many posters and charts used for teaching nutrition by the organized forces of technological society are considered critically, they can be seen to fall into three distinct groups. The first is the simplest material of propaganda – honest, well-informed and well meaning, but propaganda nevertheless – designed to drive home a single didactic point. A 'vegatabull', for instance, is a bull drawn in

145

terms of garden produce, to teach that vegetable protein supplemented by skimmed milk or dried egg is nutritionally equivalent to meat. 'Don't forget', says an elephant with a knot in its trunk, 'green vegetables keep you fit.' A picture of a child drinking milk carries the motto! 'MILK is the backbone of a young nation.' Of particular curiosity was a Jugoslav nutrition poster designed to emphasize the virtues of breast-feeding, depicting a mother in high-heeled shoes and sleek black dress putting lipstick on her face while her infant cries in a cradle with a feeding-bottle brandished in his hands. A reproving cow feeding her calf in the orthodox manner looks over the baby's head and remarks: 'Why have I to feed my own and your young as well?'

The second level of public nutrition-teaching seeks to explain as well as exhort, yet at the same time, it still retains its authoritarian attack. 'The Basic Seven . . . eat this way every day', is the slogan of the United States official teaching. The seven food categories are leafy green or yellow vegetables; citrus fruit, tomatoes and cabbage; potatoes and other vegetables and fruit; milk, cream, ice-cream; meat, poultry, fish, eggs, dried peas and beans; bread, flour, cereals (whole grain or enriched); butter and fortified margarine. All very well for the community for which it was intended, but perhaps not of general scientific validity. And the Canadian food rules, too, based on science, are applicable with advantage to a standardized community, but again empirical rather than scientific: 'These are the foods for health, eat them every day. Drink plenty of water.' Oh! The rules as at first laid down were: 'Milk – adults $\frac{1}{2}$ to 1 pint, children $1\frac{1}{2}$ pints to 1 quart. Fruit – one serving of citrus fruit or tomatoes or their juices and one serving of other fruit. Vegetables – at least one serving of potatoes, at least two servings of other vegetables, preferably leafy, green or yellow and frequently raw. Cereals and bread – one serving of whole grain cereal and at least four slices of Canadian Approved Vitamin B bread (whole wheat, brown or white) with butter. Meat and fish – one serving of meat, fish, poultry, or meat alternatives, such as beans, peas, nuts, eggs or cheese. Also use eggs and cheese at least three times a week each, and liver frequently.'

This level of teaching may be good pedagogy, but it is not science. Furthermore, it is difficult, even with the best intentions of honesty and in a true desire to improve the public health, to negotiate the blurred dividing-line between propaganda and legitimate advocacy. A case can be made undoubtedly for every United States citizen to consume milk, cream or ice-cream every day of his life; but, good advice though this may be, its absolute basis on nutritional science is questionable. Again, to eat each day citrus fruit, tomatoes or cabbage may indeed improve the citizen's health, but it also contributes to the prosperity of the Florida citrus growers. The Canadian recommendation to eat liver frequently is also good advice, but it is not an essential tenet for wellbeing; there are healthy people who eat no liver.

Traditional diets justify their wholesomeness by virtue of their having evolved through history, and by the survival of the people who ate them through their evolution. This is perhaps not a very high recommendation, but it does provide pragmatic justification. To enjoy the very substantial new benefits that modern food science can bring, demands an understanding of the nature of science by the members of the community who wish to use it if nutrition is indeed to promote health. For almost two generations, British housewives have been subjected to an educational process – in school, in welfare clinics, in women's magazines and other engines of public enlightenment. Yet in 1965 McKenzie[16] showed that, although it may be thought that women might select their purchases on the basis of the nutritional knowledge they had been taught, there are often two sets of reasons why this is not so. The first reason is that didactic, authoritarian teaching may prove to be inadequate. The people exposed to it may simply fail to understand. The second reason which McKenzie found in his study is the thesis of this book: it is that even in Western societies which believe themselves to act according to logic as illuminated by science, even then, custom, tradition, history and emotion – the last played upon by public pressures of all sorts – may be more powerful than reason. Furthermore, *price* (itself resulting from diverse social forces) is a major consideration affecting how far nutritional value influences the way in which people choose their diet. It is not surprising, therefore, that the housewives interrogated by McKenzie had confused and mainly mistaken ideas about nutrition. The freedom of a community from infectious disease has little to do with whether or not its members have been taught the principles of preventive medicine. The public health is far more dependent on efficient and well-informed public-health regulations, and sufficient wealth to provide the necessary facilities – doctors, drugs, water-supply, sewage-disposal and proper houses. It can equally be argued

[16] McKenzie, J. C., *Chem. and Ind.*, 152, 1965.

that public instruction in nutrition exerts a minimal influence on the nutritional status of a society. For nutritional health, what is wanted is again an efficient and well-informed administration, and enough money or its equivalent in the pockets of the people to enable them to buy their food.

The health of a well-to-do man in a country supplied with food owes little to the science of nutrition unless he has a scientific friend to advise him against gluttony. An ample mixed diet will supply such a man with adequate amounts of the nutrients he needs. But as he becomes progressively poorer, his choice of foods diminishes. If he is impelled by poverty to restrict his diet and that of his family; and if, furthermore, he has at the same time to live in an inadequate house without proper cooking facilities, and his wife has to go out each day to work to supplement the family income, then his diet may eventually be restricted to the least number of articles providing the basic nutrient – a source of calories – at the lowest cost. Such a diet might comprise only bread, margarine, jam and – since men undergoing hardship, wherever in the world they live, will cling to analgesic drugs to ameliorate their lot – the poor Englishman would to the end spend money on tea. In South America, he would choose coca leaves, and in Asia betel nuts.

In the wealthy technological nations of the latter part of the twentieth century, there are comparatively few people who are compelled to live on bread, margarine, jam and tea. A century ago there were more. And such people suffered from malnutrition, from deficiency of B-vitamins, vitamin A, anaemia due to lack of iron – and perhaps semi-starvation as well. Haunted by Oliver Twist and the early history of the Industrial Revolution, the British public-health authorities a hundred years later decree that thiamine (vitamin B_1) and niacin be added to white flour together with calcium and iron. Similar public-health ordinances are enforced in the United States and other countries.

Teaching the science of nutrition to ordinary members of a society who have little interest in science, exerts a minimal effect on health. People do not appear to learn the facts and principles of nutrition, and, even when they do, commonly decline to behave accordingly. Teaching nutrition to those who have influence in government may be more effective. Bread with vitamins added to it may serve to protect the health of a poor family. But adding meat or eggs, milk or vegetables to the poor family's diet would do more good than adding vitamins to their bread – and, incidentally, to the bread of everyone else, regardless of the variety and richness of their meals. The most useful thing of all those the public authorities could do might be, however, to provide the poor with a little more money with which they could buy a better diet, rather than attempting to make a poor diet more nourishing. It would be an interesting exercise to determine the present cost of preventing each separate case of malnutrition by means of enriching the bread of millions of people who had no need of the added vitamins – because their diet was adequate before the vitamins were added.

The lessons of nutrition learned by those who govern have done good. For infants and expectant mothers, the provision of milk, vitamins and minerals has been of demonstrable benefit. The schoolchildren are bigger; and, in goitrous nations, the goitres are fewer and smaller because of the iodine added to salt. But even among administrators and those who advise them, the lessons have only been half-learned. The administrators do not themselves usually understand nutritional science, and the nutritional scientists, who are doctors or biochemists, restrict themselves to medicine and biochemistry. Ethnology, anthropology, sociology, religion or tribal history, all of which have a bearing on dietary behaviour may be neglected. And if the responsible authorities – apprehensive of the cost of supplying National Dried Milk fortified with vitamin D at infant welfare clinics and school meals, or calcium tablets for pregnant women – call for the assistance of an economist, the economist they consult will himself have no knowledge of nutrition. The balance sheet is never drawn up by means of which the various ways of treating people who would otherwise be malnourished might be costed and compared. Such methods as directly dosing them, or, alternatively, changing the social organization by providing meals, or subsidizing meat, or running an advertising campaign for milk, or giving out money as children's allowances or old people's supplementary pensions – none of these things are costed in relation to the nutritional good they do.

There are three cardinal principles which must be learned if the application of nutritional science to the health of a community is to win a measure of success. The first is that health, as is apparent from the definition adopted by the World Health Organization, is a state

149

which can never be fully attained. In the end, all men die. It is a sign of how remarkable the progress of science has been in the century from the 1870s to the 1970s – since Pasteur first spelled out the nature of infectious disease – that today we expect health to be something more than the absence of the pestilences which throughout the rest of history have terrified mankind. Now, besides demanding freedom from infection and disability, the citizen of the scientific age also expects to be saved, not only from having too little to eat, or from suffering from one or other of the diseases specifically due to a nutritional deficiency, but also from minor or even unfelt effects – the existence of which is deduced from a failure of the calculated composition of the patient's diet to reach the value recommended by an expert committee. In the industrialized parts of the world, divergence from nutritional health often involves coronary heart disease and obesity as well.

But besides the difficulty of defining health in all the changing environmental pressures and strains of an organism itself passing from infancy through adolescence to maturity, senescence and death, the second matter which many people fail to grasp is that science itself never reaches finality, and never can. The schoolboy may learn that lack of insulin is the cause of diabetes, and that Banting and Best discovered how to isolate and prepare insulin for use. But this was not the end of the matter. The schoolboy, grown into a man will, if he learns what science is about, understand that although the isolation of insulin was a giant stride forward, it was only one step towards the solution of the problem of the physiological equilibrium between the supply of sugar as a source of calories and much else to the tissues, and its utilization. The history of science is one long narrative of great discoveries which are never the end of the matter, but always the beginning of a further advance towards the truth. Newton's laws subsequently corrected by Einstein, and the announcement of cortisone as a cure for rheumatoid arthritis (later shown to yield more readily to aspirin) are only two examples of how science operates. It is because science is an endless sounding of nature, that the didactic teaching of nutrition must always be ineffective.

The third reason why the power provided by nutritional science has often only a limited effect on a community's health, even when the means to which it points are available, lies in the nature of even well-informed men, whether they are scientists or administrators. All men forget; they forget the knowledge they once used, they forget that new knowledge is for ever accumulating, and – worst of all – they forget that a society is a dynamic organization which, no matter how stable it may seem, is always changing. The series of public-health measures based on the scientific discovery of the efficiency of vitamin D, led to the virtual disappearance of nutritional rickets as a common disease in Great Britain. For example, the incidence of rickets in Dundee, as measured by the admission of patients to hospital, declined steeply from 1935 onwards.[17] The first unexpected event to mar this apparently conclusive victory of science, was the appearance between 1948 and 1958 of a number of cases of rickets, not due directly to nutritional deficiency but to a genetic abnormality in the infants suffering from the disease.

The second finding to disturb the self-esteem of people who viewed with justifiable pride the welfare system of low-priced or free milk to expectant mothers, supplies of vitamin D-concentrates, and the existence of clinics, health visitors and children's allowances, was implicit in the fact that the nature of the society for which the system had been designed changed without the administrators having noticed it. Gradually reports began to appear[18] of malnutrition among immigrant children in some of the large British cities. The first of these were of nutritional rickets in Pakistani children. Later there came a general awareness that among the orderly, well administered British population there had grown up ghettos of sub-populations of coloured people.

At the end of World War II it became the fashion to boast[19] about the success with which the science of nutrition had been applied actually to bring about an improvement in the health of the British people even under the stress of war and the stringency of food shortage. In describing the steps that had been taken – the special importation of dried egg and skimmed milk from the United States, concentrated orange-juice from the Middle East, and salted cod from Iceland; the addition of chalk to flour to supplement the dietary supply of calcium; and the harvesting of rose hips to provide vitamin C[20] – in describing all this it was not customary to attribute credit to the

[17] Lowe, K. G., Mitchell, R. G., Morgan, H. G., Stewart, W. K., & Thomson, J., *Proc. Nutrition Soc.*, 21, XVIII, 1962.
[18] Ameil, G. C., & Crosbie, J. C., *Lancet*, II, 423, 1963.
[19] Pyke, M., *Brit. Med. Bull.*, 2, 228, 1944; *J. Dietet. Ass.*, 23, 90, 1947.
[20] Pyke, M., and Melville, R., *Biochem. J.*, 36, 336, 1942.

high wages and full employment, and the stimulation of a clearly-discernible national purpose for which even the most dissolute idler would come into the general social busy-ness.

The situation of the immigrant enclaves which have grown up in Great Britain in the 1950s and 1960s represents exactly the opposite influence. The British situation is indeed an excellent laboratory example of the way in which race, background, social organization and environmental stress all influence 'health'. The nutritional measures I have described apply equally to all. The immigrants from India, Pakistan, the West Indies and Africa may earn the same wages as the natives of the land. Yet the social pressures to which they are exposed are the reason why every index of public health shows their state to be worse than that of their indigenous neighbours. They are denied proper houses by public authorities and private individuals alike. The houses they are able to find cost them much more. Worst of all, the society in whose midst they live cut them off from the social-contacts without which health – 'complete physical, mental and social wellbeing' – cannot properly exist. Estranged from social contact, and deprived of any kindly human link with their neighbours, they can only form themselves into a sub-community of the larger society of the country. Those responsible for the nutrition policy of the nation, who with some success had built up a system to deal with the British problems of a generation earlier, had forgotten that the nature of a community constantly changes and that the 'vulnerable groups' of the evolving multi-racial population are consequently different from those recognized to exist when the old policy was devised. The scientific food policy was unaltered, but the society was changed. That is why rickets and under-nutrition reappeared.

CHAPTER XI

THE NATURAL HISTORY OF A POLITICAL ANIMAL

In the modern age there has grown up a new way of looking at the world and of describing reality. This is the official and scientific view (and language) in contrast with the colloquial and earthy. 'A molecular conglomerate of polymerized hexose units interlocked with the complex of linked cynnamyl alcohol units comprising the diverse lignin molecules', may be a true description of fact to a chemist; but an equally true description for a non-scientist is to call the same phenomenon a piece of wood. Similarly, it is equally true to describe conditions in countries scattered half round the world in terms of a list entitled: 'Estimated *per capita* daily calorie and protein contents of net foodstuff supplies in some developing countries as compared with the USA 1960–62',[1] as it is to go to Peru and Ceylon, Pakistan and Israel, the UAR and Uganda – all of which are included in the table – and talk to the people and try to see the conditions in which they live and the motives upon which their food habits are based.

The first language, the precise scientific talk of 'per capita daily caloric and protein content' and the official jargon about 'developing' and 'developed' countries, although it serves its purpose in dealing, at some degree of precision with a certain narrow area of meaning, may lead to error because of its very narrowness. Before this language was invented, before there were such things as 'developing nations', it was necessary to talk about Turkey and the Ottoman Empire, learn something about distant Peru, and the tribesmen of Khartoum. This approach, while less tidy and not so readily classifiable as the present United Nations language, comprised a wider area of meaning. The classification of Nigeria in the list of countries ranged in order of the calculated energy value of the 'protein content of net foodstuff supplies' gives a different kind of information about the place and its people than that obtained by a traveller who has some more direct and widely-based knowledge of the Ibo and the Yoruba who live there. And the list of vitamins and mineral values of the average

[1] FAO Production *Year Book*, Rome, 1965.

153

diet of the pigmies in the rain forests of the Congo, although it can be compared with the best scientific assessment of the nutritional requirements of the people, only gives a limited picture of the actual situation unless it is reinforced by a proper understanding of the highly-sophisticated customs by means of which the pigmies maintain themselves admirably in balance with the environment of the forest and the surrounding Negroes in the territory where they live.[2]

The science of nutrition as it is taught, and as it is very often practised, is not enough to deal with want. It is not enough to analyse a diet, to examine its content of calories and protein, the thiamine and riboflavin, niacin and biotin in it, to count the milligrams of calcium and iron, and the micrograms of copper and iodine. Nutritional surveys are two a penny. Devotedly, the nutritionists carry out clinical studies[3] to assess the incidence of protein-calorie deficiency disease among children in Haiti and Brazil, Sicily and Andhara Pradesh. But even this does not fully describe the truth.

The dietary surveys show that the United States is the best-fed country on earth.[4] The estimated *per capita* daily calories are 3,100, whereas the same survey shows that in Peru they only eat 2,230 calories. (By a statistical peculiarity, the survey shows the Japanese, too, as only getting 2,230 calories.) But how clear and vivid a picture do these seemingly precise quantitative and scientific figures give of the American situation?

'Nutritional deficiency diseases due solely to an inadequate diet have almost disappeared,' writes Dr G. A. Goldsmith of the School of Medicine, Tulane University.[5] 'The nutritional state of persons living in the United States is in general very good. We are fortunate in having an abundant and varied food supply. . . . Although primary nutritional deficiency diseases are now a rarity . . . we cannot afford to be complacent. The prevalence of obesity with its many hazards to health should concern all of us.'

These statements are true, the scientific evidence supports them. But just as a higher animal is made up of many types of living cells, the function and structure of some of which are different from those

[2] Turnbull, C. M., *The Forest People*, Simon and Schuster, New York, 1961.
[3] Patwardhan, W. N., *Proc. VI Int. Congress Nut.*, p. 310, Livingstone, Edinburgh, 1963.
[4] FAO Production *Year Book*, Rome, 1965.
[5] Goldsmith, G. A., *Nutrition Rev.*, 23, 1, 1965.

of others, yet each must be well if the being of which they are all part is to be healthy, so is a community made up of its constituent men and women who also may be of diverse types. If we turn, therefore, to a second American scientific observer, Dr Jean Mayer of the Department of Nutrition of Harvard University,[6] we find an account of evidence showing that among other United States citizens – Negro families in the Southern States – 60 per cent eat diets which are 'obviously inadequate'. 'While the calorie requirements are generally covered for all members of the family, the protein intake of the children tends to be only border-line. Calcium intakes are low in at least 25 per cent of the population, perhaps as much as 35 per cent, and iron intake is low in 12 to 15 per cent of the population; vitamin A requirements are not adequately covered in as much as 80 per cent; vitamin C intake is inadequate for much of the population, particularly the urban group, for several months of each year.'

This is one example of a group living within the main society of the nation, yet separate from it; living in a richly endowed land, yet cut off from its material wealth, and – more important than this – isolated from its social endowment as well. And incomparably more deprived even than these wretched inhabitants of the Negro colonies, are the 'migrant streams' who, year after year, like lost tribes for ever on the move, and numbering tens of thousands of Puerto Rican and other 'Whites' as well as Negro labourers and their families, follow the harvests from upstate New York to Florida. Poor, barely educated, pursuing a broken social existence, those people are of all others the most unfortunate. Their food was found[7] to consist of flour and maize grits supplemented by beans; the tails, feet, ears and neck-bones of pigs; some chicken, fish and cheese; but practically no milk. Their way of existence precluded almost any cooking. Among them were found cases of scurvy, rickets, hunger oedema, marasmus and kwashiorkor. And this in the wealthy United States.

The nutritional statistics of America give no inkling of the existence of these wretched people of the 'migrant stream'. 'It is not unusual', writes Dr Mayer, 'for migrants to follow the stream for ten or even twenty years.' Living in the wealthiest, most lavishly provisioned

[6] Mayer, J., *Nutrition Rev.*, 23, 161, 1965.
[7] Browning, R. H., & Nerthcutt, T. J., Florida Bd. of Health Monograph, No. 2, 1961.

land on earth, in which there are proportionally more doctors and nutritional experts and scientists than in any other country, their nutritional status is worse by far than that of the Congo pigmies among whom Turnbull[8] lived for more than a year. Yet the pigmies, lacking supplies of vitamin-enriched breakfast food, and the advice of the Food and Nutrition Board of the US National Research Council, enjoyed a complex and stable social system. Their co-operative methods of hunting, of building houses of branches and leaves, and, above all, their highly-organized marriage rituals and educational and legal arrangements – all these contributed to the attainment of something nearly approximating to the WHO goal of 'a state of complete physical, mental and social wellbeing'. Compared with the Congo pigmies, the health of the American citizens of the 'migrant stream' was deficient indeed. But not so much deficient in vitamin D and vitamin C, iron, protein and calories to which their rickets and scurvy, anaemia, kwashiorkor and marasmus can be attributed, as in the entire fabric of a tolerable social system. 'Serial monogamy', the coupling of men and women from one to another as the tattered migrants shift from one set of plantation hutments to the next, denies the possibility of proper human existence. The cause of death of a man killed in a traffic accident can be attributed to his skull being fractured. Alternatively, the cause of death is equally due to the restless malaise that impels him to leave the noisy vacuity of his crowded home to drive to a boxing match in the next town. Welfare workers issuing vitamin tablets to the colonies of migrating labourers will not bring them to health.

One of the most dramatic attributes of the current advance in scientific technology has been the development of means of communication. There are no parts of the world so remote that information cannot instantly be transmitted from them. There are no distances on earth so great that a representative from the United Nations cannot travel from New York, Rome, Geneva or Paris to be there the following day. And representatives from the United Nations technical agencies do in fact go. It is from their work and the statistics they collect from the governments of the territories they visit that the alarming statements about the number of people suffering from 'hunger'[9] are derived. But among the fifty or more countries who

[8] Turnbull, C. M., *The Forest People*, Simon and Schuster, New York, 1961.
[9] Sen, B. R., *State of food and agriculture 1966*, FAO, Rome, 1966.

raise many millions of pounds to support a campaign for a 'final solution' of the food problems which beset the world, and among the welfare organizations in many lands, are those who have come to understand that problems of malnutrition cannot be solved either in 'developing' or 'developed' countries, simply by supplying enough food.

Professor D. S. McLaren,[10] writing from the American University of Beirut, Lebanon, has pointed out that to say a population is suffering from 'hunger' may nowadays mean one of two different things. It may be a *medical* statement that people show signs of deficiency diseases, the diagnosis of which is confirmed when the diseases respond to dietary measures. Or it may be surveys of food consumption, a *non-medical* diagnosis based on showing that their food statistics do not come up to the official standards; this has somewhat fancifully been called 'hidden hunger'. When FAO put out their estimates that of the entire world population half to two-thirds are ill-fed, it is to 'hidden hunger' that they refer.

It must be accepted that kwashiorkor and nutritional marasmus, which form the subject of the harrowing illustrations with which Oxfam prods the consciences of charitable people, are responsible for the death of scores of thousands of children each year, and in their less severe manifestations contribute to the death of hundreds of thousands more, and blight the lives possibly of millions of others who survive. Again, it has been computed that somewhere about 20,000 children go blind every year from xerophthalmia, for lack of vitamin A in their diets; and this computation excludes China, from which no reliable information is available. In most developing countries nutritional anaemias cause much illness, and are a contributory cause of death particularly in infants and women during the child-bearing period. For the world as a whole, rickets, scurvy, beriberi and pellagra – all diseases directly due to nutritional deficiency – are less important than they once were, but still take a significant toll of victims.

But will all these nutritional diseases, manifestations of what the official organizations call 'hunger', be done away with by supplies of food purchased with all these millions of pounds of money? For the most part they are diseases of infancy and childhood, and their cause is not lack of food, but lack of knowledge or fixed behaviour based

[10] McLaren, D. S., *Lancet*, II, 86, 1963.

on one of the diverse human motives other than knowledge. 'At any moment, from Manila to Guatemala City and from Cape Town to Cairo,' wrote Professor McLaren, 'infants in their thousands are becoming sick and dying from kwashiorkor and its related syndromes – essentially due to lack of protein. The reason for their illness and death is nearly always maldistribution of protein within the family. The helpless toddler, often suddenly weaned when a new pregnancy is on the way, does not get his share. Fish, a major source of protein in Malaya, is prohibited to young children because it is believed to produce worms. Infections and infestations, often mistreated with semi-starvation diets of rice-water, barley-water, or weak tea, make his chances even poorer.'

On the green tropical island of Java, many hundreds of infants go blind and die for lack of a few milligrams of pro-vitamin A. Yet around them is all the carotene in creation – this same pro-vitamin A. Many green leaves are used for animal fodder, but are regarded as unfit for human consumption. Most south-east Asians consider rice – a commodity entirely devoid of carotene, and deficient as well in some of the essential amino acids without which kwashiorkor or some other calorie-protein deficiency disease may arise – the perfect supplementary food for infants. The structure of a human community is complex, and the inter-relationships by which its component parts are bound may be powerful and tense. An American shipload of dried egg or a team of Dutch administrators would, considered on a strictly technical – some might say 'scientific' – basis, solve the problem of xerophthalmia in Java. In fact – and science is a pragmatic system that deals with facts – neither would of itself benefit the situation in an aggressively 'free' Indonesia.

Similar instances could be multiplied of communities in which people suffer, and health is damaged, not because the means are inadequate, but rather because the knowledge or the will is lacking. Education and thought can do much, but education for whom? Every Great Power, every 'developed' nation, every liberal journalist, and half the pulpits in Christendom, shout their horror of 'hidden hunger', and hope for the time of a final solution when no one on earth will be hungry. Yet what does 'hidden hunger', which so blankets the statistical assessment of want, and confuses the issue of deficiency diseases, do to man? Does it kill, blind, or shorten life? Obesity certainly shortens life. Dr Sen, Director General of FAO,

158

says[11] that 'hidden hunger' leads to 'impaired vigour and lowered vitality and thus to idle hands', to 'prematurely ageing mothers and idle youth'. But we are not told how nutrient lack was proved to be the cause of 'impaired vigour', 'premature ageing', and 'idleness of youth'. What we *do* know is that millions of *overfed* people living in the developing countries of the world suffer the same ill-effects as ourselves, whilst their 'hidden hungry' brethren do not. Learning leads to knowledge, and hence, we must hope, to wisdom – alike for the demonstrably malnourished Javanese, to the Dutch administrators who know well that vitamins must take their place in the balance with political autonomy for Indonesia, both being components of the human situation, and for Dr Sen as well.

In Java the children suffer from malnutrition because the society of which they are a part lacks the knowledge of the vitamin A-activity in the herbage around them. In the United States, pockets of the population are poor and hungry because the rich society of which *they* form a part does not know that they exist. Louis Heron[12] quotes a senior medical officer of one of the Great Society programmes as saying 'we know more about nutrition in Pakistan than we do in the United States'. Using the official Government statistics and the official Government definition of 'poverty', which carries within it the inherent implication (as did Rowntree's, 'poverty line' in York in 1899) of inevitable hunger, the investigators of the Citizens Crusade[13] related the number of 'poor' people to the number receiving any relief from official programmes to supply the needy with food. In Connecticut, the second richest state in the Union, 236,220 people were found officially classified as 'poor'; only 4,945 were on the lists of those receiving free or cheap food. In South Carolina, 715,778 were 'poor', 10,878 were given help, and 17 out of 20 countries investigated had no programme of help at all. In the 15 southern and border states, more than 3 million 'poor' people were found to whom no state welfare programme was available; of 7 million others officially categorized as 'poor' and by definition in need of aid, aid was provided for 1 million.

---

[11] Browning, R. H., & Nerthcutt, T. J., Florida Bd. of Health Monograph, No. 2, 1961.

[12] Heron, L., *The Observer*, London, 20 Jun. 1967.

[13] *Rept. of the Citizens Crusade against Poverty*, Ford Foundation and CIO, 1967.

Nutritional knowledge, for lack of which children may go blind and die, concerns the role of vitamin A and xerophthalmia. But no community *wants* children to suffer from malnutrition. When they do, the knowledge lacking may be partly that of the biochemical mechanism of vitamin A, and partly of the social mechanism which moves, for instance, the Javanese community to live as it does. Or, where eight or nine million Americans are poor and underfed, the knowledge lacking – certainly not that of nutritional science as taught at Harvard – may be of the principles by which the behaviour of a community of men, some white, some black, some Puerto Rican, is determined. And of how to learn to see the condition of one's own body-politic, even though not all of it is healthy.

The beneficial effects of nutritional science, indeed of the whole of modern medicine and public health, have been clear and dramatic. There has, however, been a serious danger of overestimating the capabilities of science to apply its own knowledge – as in the failure of the Javanese to use the green leaves from their countryside, and the Americans to use the wealth from their industry. The behaviour of a society, and particularly its understanding of its true wealth, are every bit as important as factors conducive to health as is nutritional or scientific knowledge. Dr Harald Frederiksen, medical director of the Public Health Service of the US Office of Technical Co-operation and Research, has presented cogent evidence[14] to show that the beneficial effects of a scientific nutrition-policy and an up-to-date health service are achieved, not by themselves, but hand in hand with other improvements in the levels of living.

Dazzled by the remarkable discoveries in nutrition and medicine, nutritionists and public-health workers are inclined to believe that they alone hold the keys to a healthy society. Many intelligent administrators also come to believe that these aspects of applied biochemistry possess such powerful magical powers that, if the most up-to-date findings of science are applied to backward societies, their people will live so long that their final state may be worse than their first. It is sometimes said that, far from benefiting from science, they will be pushed into a 'Malthusian trap'.[15] Too many lives will be saved, so that all will starve. The facts, however, are different.

In 1946 and 1947, large areas of Ceylon were sprayed with DDT to

[14] Frederiksen, H., *US Publ. Hlth. Rep.*, Wash., 81, 715, 1966.
[15] Cipolla, C. M., *The economic history of world population*, Penguin, 1964.

destroy the malaria-bearing mosquito. This application of modern science was effective, and, where it was done, malaria was virtually stamped out. In these same years, the death rate in Ceylon as a whole fell from 20 to 14 per 1,000. 'The death rate in Ceylon was cut in half in less than a decade,' wrote an expert committee of the US National Academy of Sciences.[16] '. . . The result of a precipitous decline in mortality while the birth rate remains essentially unchanged is, of course, a very rapid acceleration in population growth . . . economic progress will eventually be stopped and reversed unless the birth rate declines or the death rate increases.' It was implied that one of the principal factors leading to this state of affairs was the application of science in the form of 'the use of residual insecticides to provide effective protection against malaria at a cost of no more than 25 cents *per capita* per annum'. The facts of the matter were, however, that the economy of Ceylon had been improving, and the standard of living of the people rising, *before* the malaria-suppression campaign was begun. Furthermore, the reduction in mortality was just as spectacular in those parts of the country where no insecticides were used as in the parts which were sprayed.[17]

The situation in Mauritius told the same story. The dramatic reduction in the death rate – from 30 per 1,000 in 1946, to 20 per 1,000 in 1947 – was again attributed primarily to the spraying of insecticides. But when the situation was examined in more detail, it was found that when the island was prosperous and sugar production – sugar is virtually the sole export – was high, the death rate tended to fall. This supports the conclusion that health is a concomitant of a combination of social factors; many of these can be expressed in the omnibus terms 'economic prosperity', some of them can be described as 'social harmony' or 'national self-respect' or 'freedom', although among others must undoubtedly be included scientific understanding and technical ability. But this last is not the whole. In Mauritius, while the dramatic drop in death rate occurred between 1946 and 1947, when the *per capita* sugar production went up from around 600 kilos to 900 kilos, the spraying campaign to destroy the mosquitoes was only started in 1949!

Science can be argued to benefit the health of a community when it is used by that community to increase real wealth. When it is applied

[16] US Nat. Acad. Sci., Pub. 1091, Wash, 1963.
[17] Frederiksen, H., US *Pub. Health Rep.*, Wash., 75, 865, 1960.

from without as gifts of dried milk or fish flour, DDT or penicillin, vitamin tablets or contraceptive pills, its value is limited. A mission, organized by the International Bank for Reconstruction and Development (impressed like so many other Western observers by the prestige of science), issued a report[18] about the effect of the campaign to spray all the houses in British Guiana with DDT. 'The disappearance of malaria,' they wrote, 'brought about a sharp fall in the death rate. . . . In particular, infant mortality showed a striking decrease from 110·7 per 1,000 live births in 1940–45 to 81·8 in 1946–51.' Once again, however, this facile deduction does not stand up to scrutiny. Dr Frederiksen[19] examined the British Guiana infant mortality rates from 1930 to 1960. Considerable fluctuations occurred from year to year, but when the figures were plotted and a curve drawn, the trend, as indicated by the 'least-square' line, was found to be constant. The mean value for 1930 was 170 deaths per 1,000 live births; for 1935, 1940 and 1945 the values were 150, 125 and 100. In 1947 and 1948 the spraying which so impressed the International Bank was done. And in 1950, 1955 and 1960 the steady fall in infant mortality continued with mean values of 85, 70 and 60. Medical science, food science, biological science (giving contraceptive pills), toxicological science (destroying pests), and military science (killing enemies), are all in their way important and powerful. But each contributes only a part to any social change. The real knowledge by which progress is to be made towards that 'complete mental physical and social wellbeing' which the United Nations – and indeed, before them, every dreamer who has conceived a Utopia for his nation – has hazily defined as 'health', is the understanding of human behaviour.

Even in a technologically advanced and wealthy country organized as a corporate human society with an efficient central government broadly acceptable to all its members, although a great deal can be done by the application of scientific knowledge to the nutritional state of the population, there is a limit. We have already seen that, even after thirty years of signally successful British nutritional planning, rickets may appear in Dundee. In the United States the numbers of those who are malnourished may be counted in millions.

[18] International Bank for Reconstruction and Development, *The economic development of British Guiana*, Johns Hopkins Press, 1953.
[19] Cipolla, C. M., *The economic history of world population*, Penguin, 1964.

These are two of the wealthy nations of the world; what then must be the state of poor countries? Being poor, their food supplies are less assured; they come mainly from the country's own resources, where they are vulnerable to a bad harvest; or, when food is purchased, the money to buy it is often derived from the sale of a single primary product which itself is at the mercy of weather, uncontrollable fluctuations in market price, or, at worst, technological obsolescence. Wealth, scientific knowledge and a recognition of the unitary nature of the whole human race, have led to the remarkable growth of international benevolence, much of which has grown up since World War II, which has been manifest as the various international aid programmes. But when we find the nutritional measures taken by sophisticated, close-knit states such as America and Britain failing to achieve full success, we are surely overestimating both the benevolence, and the knowledge of food science and anthropology alike, if we imagine that – by taking thought – we can solve the problem of so-called developing countries over which we have no authority to impose such scientific measures as we may devise.

The 'scientific' attack on world malnutrition is lacking in three respects. First of all, knowledge of the biochemistry of nutrition, detailed and effective though it has become in the last two decades, is ineffective without equally complete scientific knowledge of human ecology – that is, how men behave in harmony or in competition with other members of their colony, in relation to the climate, the land, the cities they live in, and all the environmental paraphernalia of twentieth-century life. The second area of ignorance, which those who plan to apply nutritional knowledge to practical affairs must at least recognize, is economics. The Affluent Society is not fully under the intellectual control of those who run it, nor are all its citizens affluent. Communities will continue to suffer from kwashiorkor, due to inadequate supplies of protein for young children, even if welfare organizations set up a factory to make fish flour, or lay out plantations of groundnuts, should the indigenous population find it more profitable to sell the fish flour and the groundnuts than to eat them. And the third reason why science of itself is not enough is that international aid may be twisted by the unclear motives of the donors.

When in the middle of the nineteenth century 'advanced' countries began to adopt science as one of the basic philosophical principles upon which society should be run, Darwin's ideas were seriously taken to apply to social conduct. The principles of evolution were often expressed as the 'survival of the fittest'. Man had only achieved his predominant position as head of creation because he was fit to dominate and, if he wished, exterminate any other species. Within the community of mankind, therefore, it could equally aptly be argued that rich successful men, and powerful and dominant trading-nations, were successful, powerful and dominant because they were fitter than the others. A corollary of this argument was, that to help poor, weak and unsuccessful people was foolish, unscientific and likely to hold back the progress of human evolution. As the nineteenth century gave way to the twentieth, this fundamental doctrine was gradually modified until in almost all educated communities – even the United States, where pure scientific thinking had been deeply entrenched – the idea of a welfare state emerged, and from this grew the present notion of the welfare world supported by the global association of the United Nations.

But parallel with the accepted principle that it was the duty of rich nations to give aid to poor ones, there grew up an equally loudly asserted doctrine that every nation, no matter how small, poor, ignorant and incompetent, had a right to its own absolute freedom to run its own affairs. These two tenets were given practical support by very large subventions of aid by the donor nations. For example, in 1944 the official aid expenditure of the United States was 3,534 million dollars, that of France 841 million dollars, and those of Great Britain and Germany 490 and 460 million dollars respectively.[20]

International aid comprises money, goods, food and technical advice. The Food and Agriculture Organization and the World Health Organization of the United Nations, as I have already mentioned, carry out nutritional and medical surveys in developing nations all over the world. The principal nations contributing aid, notably the United States, France, Great Britain and Germany, also provide technical and administrative advisers and, in addition, there are numerous foundations and charitable and religious organizations which go out from Western technological nations to advise and help those whom they consider to be less fortunate than themselves. Yet the philosophical observer of this massive deployment of dynamic

[20] Organization of Economic Co-operation and Development, Development Assembly Efforts and Policies, Rev. 1965.

164

benevolence may well ask whether it achieves the ends for which it is devised. We have already seen from Chapter IV that the mercenary Western ethic may, by breaking up an existing closely-knit social system, do more harm than good; and, by accustoming a community to the sophisticated products of Western technology, pauperize the people whom it was intended to help.

Considerable thought has been given to the effectiveness of aid as a means of achieving the economic development and hence, presumably, the improved nutritional status, of poor countries.[21] The results of such reflections show that effectiveness is uneven and the purposes for which the aid is given diverse. The French and the Americans are clear on two matters. The first is that they know better than the recipients what is good for them. Secondly, these two nations are candidly aware that, no matter how kindly their feelings are towards the 'have-not' nations, the reason for disbursing men and treasure in the form of aid is basically to benefit France and America. To a French official it is 'obvious' that by giving aid to a developing nation France is exerting influence. The American nutritionist, R. R. Williams, Chairman of the Williams-Waterman Fund for the Combat of Dietary Diseases, found nothing incongruous in concluding an article on 'Chemistry as a supplement to agriculture in meeting the world's food needs'[22] with the words: 'Manufacturing chemistry can ultimately aid agriculture greatly by producing synthetically and selectively those essential components of food which are required in minor amounts. . . . The dominant peoples in whose hands now reside the scientific knowledge and technology of present-day earth are already outnumbered manyfold by the dark-skinned races in need of our help. If we do not aid them, communism will surely attempt to do so and will use these people as cannon fodder to destroy us.'

Equally well-meaning, with equal knowledge of science, and fully as single-minded, the Soviet Union also has launched out into a massive programme of loans and foreign aid. It has been estimated[23] that between 1954 and 1965 Soviet credits and grants extended to developing countries amounted to some $5,000 m. About 41 per cent of this

[21] Rept. of int. conf. of Ditchley Foundation and Overseas Development Inst., *Effective Aid*, ODI, London, 1966.
[22] Williams, R. R., *Amer. Sci.*, 44, 317, 1956.
[23] *The Times*, p. 8, London, 26 Sep. 1967.

was spent in the Middle East, partly, no doubt, to improve the nutritional status of the Arab nations, but partly for reasons similar to those expressed by the Chairman of Williams-Waterman Fund for the Combat of Dietary Diseases.

'Reflecting on his voyages to Polynesia in the late eighteenth century, Captain Cook later wrote that "It would have been better for these people never to have known us" . . . Even when acting with the best of intentions, Americans, like other Western peoples who have carried their civilizations abroad, have had something of the same fatal impact on smaller nations that European explorers had on the Tahitians and the native Australians.'[24] Scientists going into the 'hungry' countries to bring the benefits of nutritional science can deploy valuable knowledge provided they appreciate that they do not possess the whole of wisdom. In August 1967, the Fourth Rehovoth Conference held in Israel was devoted to health problems in developing States. The main theme running through the conference was that in planning health services and medical education, the new countries must not copy the patterns of the old – patterns which many of the old 'developed' nations themselves now realize to be far from ideal in the modern world. In an address which to a large degree summarizes the intent of this book, Dr M. G. Candau, director-general of the World Health Organization,[25] made a plea for an ecological approach in which man would be viewed as inseparable from his environment, his ancestry and his culture; and he called on countries that had emerged from colonialism to free themselves also from 'technological colonialism'. For one thing, the nutritional scientists, trained in biochemistry, physiology, food chemistry and clinical medicine, who come to colonize them, do not always know enough to achieve what they set out to do. McGonigle[26] years ago set out to help the poor, undernourished slum-dwellers of Stockton-on-Tees. His nutritional knowledge was in advance of his generation, his clinical acumen was outstanding, his science impeccable and his drive and force of character untiring. Yet when his work was done, and the unfortunate people of the town were rehoused in fine, new, sanitary dwellings, their health deteriorated and the death rate rose. The rents of their

[24] Fulbright, J. W., *The Arrogance of Power*, Cape, London, 1967.
[25] *Lancet*, II, 551, 1967.
[26] McGonigle, G. C. A., and Kirby, L., *Poverty and Public Health*, London, 1936.

166

new houses were higher than those of the squalid tenements they had lived in before.

Molecular biology has been a potent intellectual force. As we have seen, beri-beri was once a disease which scourged the East. It decimated the Japanese Navy; its victims in the Philippines, in Indonesia, Malaya, and Central America were numbered in tens of thousands; for want of a few grams of thiamine – obtainable today by the ton – a British army was compelled to surrender to the Turks at Kut-el-Amara.[27] The highly technical discovery of Lohmann and Schuster in 1937[28] that a diphosphate ester of vitamin B_1 functions as the co-enzyme, cocarboxylase – lacking which pyruvic acid accumulates in the tissues and by its toxic effect causes the symptoms of beri-beri leading swiftly, if not relieved, to death – was the key to the relief of mankind from beri-beri. Without this scientific knowledge, British generals, Japanese admirals and the Dutch administrators of the Orient were helpless. But because he possesses it, the nutritional scientist is not equipped to solve the problems of developing nations abroad, nor even those of Stockton-on-Tees at home. It can now quite clearly be seen that governments and their administrators, charitable organizations and missionaries, and the special agencies of the great United Nations alike, need a new kind of approach to the situations with which they set out to deal. Nutrition based, as it has been, on molecular biology is not enough: 'para-nutrition' is required.

Para-nutrition must incorporate an understanding of the reasons behind men's food fallacies. Essentially it deals with food, nutrition and eating in the context of human ecology. A man equipped to deal with para-nutritional problems must be something more than an inspired amateur; he needs to have at his command, either in his own head or in those of the technical advisers he gathers around him, a proper knowledge of nutrition and of economics, agriculture and the dozen or more of scientific disciplines which apply to the complexity of the scientific age in the twentieth century. But even to appreciate the usefulness of these sciences, and the depth of scholarship which they now provide, is not enough. The Admirable Crichton whom we now need to cope with the poor and starving people of the modern world must also appreciate the limitation of science. The molecular biologist may rightly understand the nature of DNA, the molecule

[27] Heher, C., *Mesopotamia Commission Rept.*, Appendix III, 1917.
[28] Lohmann, K., and Schuster, P., *Naturwissenschaften*, 25, 26, 1937.

controlling genetical inheritance, without being in the least able to arrange to manufacture a Michelangelo, or, indeed, without possessing any very clear idea about what sort of person he would choose were he able to produce such a person at will. The para-nutritionist may understand the factors causing malnutrition in Egypt – lack of B-vitamins, lack of calories, intestinal worms, lack of industrial development, and hatred of Israel – without fully knowing how to remedy the situation.

The flowering of scientific discovery and its application to practical affairs have constituted one of the major revolutions in the narrative of man. But the revolution has happened and is beginning to dwindle into the perspective of history. It remains to use wisely what it has achieved.

Medicine is a science-using technology. Medical education therefore aims to produce men educated in science and capable of using it to benefit the health of their patients; it is not designed to produce either scientists on the one hand or, on the other, educated men who know what medicine is about, but without the ability to heal. It has recently been recognized that medical education has been acquiring two opposite kinds of heresy.[29] First, the student is being taught too much science by teachers impatient of the untidy needs of the real emergencies of ill and frightened people: if he listens he becomes intolerant of individual patients; if he does not, he becomes contemptuous of science. The second heresy is, therefore, in reaction, the 'pastoral fallacy'. This implies that devotion to his flock is the doctor's main purpose; yet without the science-based technology it has little virtue. For the doctor, the remedy proposed is to integrate science into his whole training instead of keeping it separate. This simple prescription is equally applicable to any modern Joseph called by his conscience or by Pharaoh to administer a Land of Egypt's food supply through the lean years.

[29] Dornhorst, A. C., and Hunter, A., *Lancet*, II, 666, 1967.

INDEX

INDEX

Abies balsamea, source of 'juvenile hormone', 113
abstinence, relation to moral virtues, 13, 50
accessory food factors, discovery and identification, 3
Accum, Friedrich, and white bread abuses, 73
additives, public attitude to their use, 114; pursuit of safety, 115–18; pharmacological study of, 117–18; dangers from unintentional use, 118; Expert Commission on, 127; principles justifying their use, 131
affluence, and choice of food, 41
affluent society, limited application, 163
Aflatoxin, in contaminated groundnuts, 111–12; carcinogenic toxicity, 111–12; does it affect man?, 112
Africa, use of dogflesh, 13; dietary beliefs of Zulus, 28–9; magical beliefs, 31, 32; racial variations in diet, 39, 43; beer-drinking, 43–6; food production, 82, 83; and Codex Alimentarius Commission, 135
agriculture, belief in technological advances, 58; to be replaced by 'agri-business', 122
alcohol, and social behaviour, 46
Allinson, T. R., 74
aluminium, use of for cooking pans, 95–6; said to cause cancer, 95
America, Latin, food production, 82, 83; draft code for Codex Alimentarius, 130
anaemia, nutritional, 156, 157
animal life, extinction of species by food technology, 122
Arabs, magical beliefs, 23
Aspergillus flavus, in contaminated groundnuts, 111–12

Astwood, E. B., and hyperthyroidism, 104
Australia, 'kangaroo man', 21; aboriginal belief in sorcery, 35; use of insects for food, 42, 43; effect of white men on its habitat, 60
Austwick, P. K. C., and poisonous groundnuts, 111
avocados, toxic content, 105–6

bachelor scurvy, 34
Bantu people, magical beliefs concerning food, 29, 30; dietary customs, 44–5; high incidence of liver tumours, 112
baptism, 21
Beaton, G. H., and McHenry, E. W., *Nutrition,* 83
'benefit/risk ratio', 120
beri-beri, vitamin deficiency disease, 4, 74, 86, 87, 97, 144, 157; frame of mind induced by, 87; discovery of cure for, 167
Betts, Charles T., condemnation of aluminium, 95
Bible, references to magical foods, 22; food prohibitions, 57–8; effect on health of different diets, 70
biology, new approach to its teaching, 144–5
Blackwell, B., and Womack, A. M., and tyramine in cheese, 108
Bloch, C. E., xerophthalmia in children, 3
Blumenthal, C., and aluminium cooking vessels, 96
Bodenheimer, F. S., and insects as food, 40–1, 42, 43
bread, Graham and, 14–15; position in religious liturgy, 72, 73; alleged superiority of brown over white, 72–7; discovery of vitamins and, 74; analytical arguments, 74–5;

bread – *continued*
  experiments concerning, 76–7; use of flour additives, 117
British Guiana, fall in death rate, 162
British Medical Association, 4, 85; Committee on Nutrition, 90
British Medical Research Council, 139; experiment on restricted diet, 91
broad beans, toxic reaction, 107–8
Bryant, A. T., and Kaffir-beer, 43–4

caffeine, 46, 47–8
Camboué, Fr R. P., and locust-eating, 42–3
Canadian Food Rules, 146
Candau, M. G., plea for an ecological approach to health, 166
canning, misunderstandings concerning, 81
Cannon, W. B., and voodooism, 33, 34
caramel, industrial manufacture, 135–6
Cassel, John, use of history to combat food prejudice, 28–9, 30
caste, and diet, 38
Ceylon, fall in death rate, 160–1
cheese, 125, 126; toxic component, 108–9
China, use of dogflesh, 13; insect-eating, 42
Christianity, victory over paganism; 61; an anthropocentric religion, 61–2, 63, 67; destruction of sacred groves, 62–3, 67
cigarette-manufacturers, and lung cancer, 93
Citizens Crusade, classification of 'poor' people, 159
Codex Alimentarius Commission, setting up, 123, 126; its purpose, 123–4, 126; executive committee, 126; work of the Commission, 127–8; statement of general principles, 128–30; absorption in generalities, 129; Latin-American draft code, 130; diversity of details considered, 131–3; secondary purpose, 135; and a Co-ordinating Committee for Africa, 135; inherent dangers, 136

cod-liver oil, 2–3
Codrington, R. H., *Melanesians*, 21
Coles, William, and Doctrine of Signatures, 25
colonialism, technological, dangers of, 166–7
conservation, modern acceptance, 67–8
cooking utensils, aluminium, 95–6
Cooper, R. M. Le Hunte, condemnation of aluminium, 95–6
coronary heart disease, and fat consumption, 97–8; and coumarin, 110
Corry Mann, H. C., 143
coumarin, as a flavouring agent, 109; and coronary thrombosis, 110
Crandon, J. H., and vitamin C-deficiency, 4
Culpeper, Nicholas, 25
custom, effect on human behaviour, 37; and choice of food, 38, 40, 43; a characteristic of the group, 43; importance to human welfare, 47–8; and new food habits, 50

Dahomey, the, 56
Darwin, Charles Robert, 49; application of 'survival of the fittest' to mankind, 164
DDT, its ubiquitousness, 118–19; and a falling death rate, 160–1, 162
death, caused by magic, 33, 34, 36
death rate, relation to 'poverty line', 6
Dick, O. L., *Brief Lives*, 71–2
diet, religious beliefs and, 12; attribution of moral virtues to, 13; racial variations, 37–9; twentieth century limitations, 40; general factors influencing, 40 *ff.*; effect of science and technology on, 51; effect on health of differing types, 70; difficulties of finding out, 83, 84; determination of an optimum amount, 138; effect on life span, 141; justification of traditional ones, 147; sciences concerned with, 149
dietetics, original confusion, 94
diseases, germ theory of, 1; caused by vitamin deficiency, 3–4, 86, 156; and certain foods, 12; caused by dietary deficiency, 39; carried by

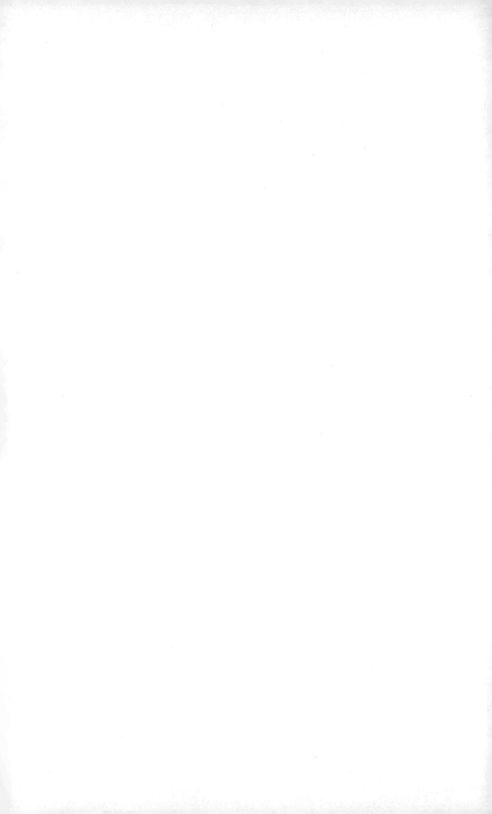